A HANDBOOK FOR CANADIANS OVER FIFTY

SENIOR SIDE OF LIVING

IRENE CRAWFORD

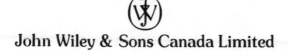

John Wiley & Sons Canada Limited

Personal Library, Publishers
Suite 539, 17 Queen Street East
Toronto, Canada M5C 1P9

Publisher: Glenn Edward Witmer
Editor: Richard Prybyzerski
Design: First Image
Cover Photographs: Lynda Middleton
Typesetting: Pickwick Typesetting Limited

A Personal Library publication
produced exclusively for
John Wiley and Sons Canada Limited
22 Worcester Road, Rexdale, Ontario
M9W 1L1

A special thanks to the London Free Press.

Canadian Cataloguing in Publication Data

Crawford, Irene, 1927-
  Senior SIDE OF LIVING

Includes index.
ISBN 0-471-99833-8

1. Aged.   2. Old age.   I. Title.

HQ1061.C73   301.43'5   C79-094634-3

Printed and bound in Canada

To Mom

CONTENTS

This Aging Process

Aging is a journey we must all take, yet of all things that determine a person's age, birthdays are the least important. Age is a span of life, and old age, a time when we look back, a time when we accept what is, and a time when we assess the future.

The quality of our life in our future years will be governed by three things: health, financial status and attitude. Of the three, attitude is the most important. How do we see ourselves? How do we feel about this aging process? Are we going to fight it, or are we going to accept it?

Aging is not just something that happens to us; it is a natural and universal process. There is no fountain of youth. Our society says we are senior citizens at age 65. Yet Bulwer-Lytton, the nineteenth century English novelist, said, "It is not by the gray of the hair that one knows the age of the heart." Often there is a vast difference between chronological and physiological age.

Many of the problems of aging are in our minds. If we think we are old, we are old. If we think we can't

4

be productive, we can't produce. In our later years, the quality of our lives will be governed by what we *can* do, not by what we can't do!

In our younger years, we read to our children the story of the little train who succeeded in climbing up a big hill by repeating:

> I think I can,
> I think I can,
> I know I can,
> I can!

This must be our attitude toward aging; we must be positive about growing old.

Dr. Ronald Cape, former consultant and physician in geriatric medicine at the South Birmingham Group of Hospitals in Birmingham, England, and now professor and co-ordinator of geriatric medicine at the University of Western Ontario in Canada, says, "It is better to face the fact of aging than to try to blot it out or disguise it. We should make the most of it." Good figures, handsome faces and straight backs are for a different time; there is no tragedy in the physical transformation of our bodies.

Although the hectic pace of middle age may slow to a walk, maybe even a crawl, the quality of our lives need not deteriorate. Each age has its own joys, its own sorrows, its own challenges. Now we must look for the inner beauties and revel in them.

For years we have been brainwashed into believing nothing good can come of aging. Even literature and art have given us a false impression of oldness. Did you know that Whistler's Mother was only 44 when she sat for that famous portrait? She looked decades older.

In Ancient Greece, the young were the aged— their life span was 18 years. The Romans improved the standard of living a little: their seniors reached old age at 22. Now, with improvements in the fields of health, retirement and finance, our life span has increased more than three-and-a-half fold. Today's man can expect to live until he is 79; his wife's life expectancy is 82.

Inactivity, both mental and physical, are the greatest saboteurs of productive aging. "You don't lose all your marbles the day you become 65," said Sister St. Michael Guinan, founder of the Canadian Institute of Religion and Gerontology, and considered one of Canada's foremost authorities on aging. "People keep telling me you can't teach an old dog new tricks, but I tell them no one yet has told the dog, and he just goes on learning." Sister St. Michael is in her late eighties and still going strong, writing, speaking at workshops and seminars, breaking new ground for seniors.

Unless disease strikes, mental powers don't just slip away. Many seniors feel just because they qualify for Old Age Security, they are ready for the rocking chair. This is utter nonsense. People are the same at 65 as they were at 58; true, they now have a few more wrinkles, their hair is a little whiter, but inwardly they are just the same. Only the facade has changed.

Actually, the human body matures in 25 to 30 years; after that, it minutely shrinks. We do not age uniformly; like a boat, some parts break down before others. But our bodies have wonderful resources and they bounce back, although at a slower pace. By using these resources to their fullest potential, we can still have a life that is meaningful, that has purpose and quality.

Seniors are no longer a forgotten minority; they are an active, clear thinking, independent segment of our society, but, unfortunately, the experience of aging has changed faster than our understanding of it.

To help correct this dearth of knowledge, universities and colleges across the United States and Canada are offering courses in gerontology and other subjects related to the aging process. They are delving into such subjects as work and leisure, congenital and sexual functioning, personality development, investment and pensions and current biological theories on aging.

However, it is not just seniors who need to be educated. Society, too, must learn to realize that after 65, life does have purpose. One senior vehemently voiced his opposition this way: "When one reaches that so-called magical age, we are treated as though we are momentarily going to be entering the heavenly gates. It is a distorted, bovinely stupid attitude."

Seniors don't need to add years to life—they need to add life to years. People who retain a zest for living are not put out to pasture. They can remain alert and active well into their 70s and 80s and often their 90s.

Aging is not a disease; it is a natural progression from one season of life to another. It is true seniors are going to face traumatic experiences: loss of work due to retirement or the phasing out of one's job, loss of home, loss of health, and most traumatic of all—loss of spouse. Those seniors who coped successfully with the last 65 years or more, will cope now; they are strong, their lives have been tempered with war and depression, sickness and sorrow.

Four out of five seniors will live out their lives in their own homes, will retain full independence and reasonably good health. Less than 4 per cent will be institutionalized. For them, recollections of the past will go hand in hand with the present and future. But no matter what the age, life is still precious. That is a fact of life the young easily forget or misunderstand, yet that fact lies at the centre of all efforts to improve the quality of life for the elderly. To know why, we must listen to the voices of the elderly and learn from their experience. One woman in a nursing home on the eve of her 90th birthday summed it up this way: "'Isn't it wonderful; you're going to be 90 tomorrow.' That's what people have been saying to me all day. Wonderful? Well, let me tell you about being old; it's good and it's bad.

"The truth is everyone knows you're old long before you do. Just like that morning five years ago when my daughters came to my house. 'Mother, you can't look after yourself any more, and we're too busy to look in on you every day. Besides, the doctor says it's best if you go into a nursing home.'

"I didn't believe them, but here I am. For a long time, when they came to visit, I wanted to beg, 'Please take me home. Please!' But I never begged when I was young, and I'm certainly not going to beg now that I'm old. I have my pride; it is one of the few things I do have left.

"I know I am going to die—everyone dies—it is just part of the cycle, but I want to die in my own bed, in my own home, with familiar things around me, with someone who loves me holding my hand.

Even here in the nursing home life is precious; there is love here and kindness, and I'm happy. I know I complain a lot; that's because I'm often uncomfortable, and sometimes very afraid. I have climbed my mountains, and pushed through a good many valleys; now there is just one valley left, and the path is so dark.

"I don't want to die among strangers, people who just see the outside of me, my wrinkled, prune-like body, bony and ugly. I want people to see me as I used to be, pretty, laughing, happy, with my cheeks 'the color of peach blush,' my husband used to say, not this sallow grey color.

"'She's 89, she'll be 90 tomorrow, but poor dear, her mind wanders,' my relatives say. I know I wander; there are so many years back there, so many pleasant memories—ahead, a white sheet over my face, a wreath on my coffin, so why shouldn't I dwell in the past?

"Sometimes I don't want to eat. 'Just being ornery,' the nurse likes to say. One of the joys of my life is evening the score with her, and I do get the chance once in a while. 'Perfectly good food, no reason she can't eat it,' the nurse complains to her helper, and she's right. But today's menu is the same as last week's menu.

"Remember how I used to cook cauliflower and cover it with a rich cheese sauce? And there was the wild raspberry jam I used to make. Because I'm 89, no one knows how I long for a piece of home-made lemon pie or a sip of ice-cold apple cider.

"There are mornings when I wake up just plain tired. Instead of resting, I must get washed, dressed, sit in my chair, eat my breakfast, take my exercise, then repeat part of the process two more times the same day. 'How do you expect to sleep tonight if you sleep all day?' someone prods me.

"Resting my eyes is not sleeping. For a while I escape from these surroundings, back into the world of laughing children (I had five) and a husband who loved me. I escape to the world where there are picnics at the side of a river; where there was joy in work, when you could taste the harvest.

"When I open my eyes, all I see that really belongs to me is a chair and a TV and an old flower stand, and I hate them. They remind me that this is all that is left of my life, and I want to shut my eyes again.

9

"Sometimes in the night I have an 'accident,' and the nurse's aide says, 'Shame! You know better than that. Just for being so naughty, I'm going to let you lie in that until morning.' She pats me on the head like I was a child.

"How can I tell someone like that that I was on my way to the outhouse, but the path was too long—and this just happened. When my babies were small, I never let them lie in their wet. I kept them dry and fresh, powdering their little bottoms with corn starch and boracic acid; we didn't have fancy commercial powders.

"And I smell so. Even after they put on fresh sheets and pillow cases, and clean things for me. Yesterday I spilled some milk on my dressing gown; it's gone sour. I drool and my wobbly hands just can't seem to wipe it away. How can I stand myself?

"Yesterday they wheeled away the patient in the next bed. I cried. Not because she wasn't coming back, but because I knew she had found the peace she sought.

"Now tomorrow is my birthday and I'll be 90. My family will come and friends will visit, and the staff will give me a party and everyone will say, 'Isn't it wonderful?' But how would you like to be me?"

How would you like to be me . . . this "me" will be you in the future. We might not like it, we might fight against it, but it is part of the natural progression. How we accept this progression of time will govern the quality of our remaining years, because aging is a journey we must all take.

Our Heritage From the Past

The characters of seniors today have been molded and tempered by the past. So that we can improve the quality of life in our later years, we must understand where we have been in order to know where we are going.

And where we have been hasn't always been that good, although there was the gentleness of the early 1900s and the fun of the free-wheeling Roaring Twenties; to temper the frivolity, there was the horror of World War I and the Great Depression.

These were the times in which today's seniors were born, the times of their youth, the times that shaped their characters.

As the Depression swept like a black shroud over North America, people learned to fight for jobs; proud men learned to beg, and women who had never sewn on a button learned to "make do." Children wore hand-me-downs and went barefoot until snow. People learned to live off the land; their only meat was wild rabbit, or fish from a nearby stream.

Telephones were here to stay, but many who had them became had-nots when they couldn't pay their bills. Most homes had electricity, but those with overdue accounts saw their supply cut, and wick lamps with their dangling prisms came out of the closets.

Some families were broken apart; husbands deserted wives and children; others were knit closer by hardship and poverty. Seniors of today like to tell about the past, because it was so much a part of their growing-up years.

"We rented a farm; the one we owned was sold for the $1800 mortgage that was called. The land was poor, mostly sand, and a few days after we planted our crops, the winds came, and our seed ended up in the neighbor's field. That was a bad year for us—no harvest. Our only income came from the butter Mother churned and sold door to door.

"When winter came, our taxes had still not been paid. Just to keep a roof over our heads Mother and Dad went to the bush, and Mother learned to pull her weight on the end of a cross-cut saw.

"Bankruptcies were common, and mother begged father to declare ourselves broke. His sister (all I remember about her was her long scrawny neck) intervened; our name was a proud name; we could not drag it into the courts, she said.

"At least we would have gotten out from under our mountain of debts. When a farmer declared bankruptcy, he was allowed a team of horses, a cow, a dozen or so chickens, plus one piece of necessary machinery such as a plow, harrows and wagon, and of course his household furnishings. By taking this route, in time we could have landed back on our feet, but until the day he died, Dad was never free of debt. He suffered out the Depression and it almost killed him; worse, it broke his spirit."

12

The Depression was the era of make-do—make-do with what you had. One senior recalled the wonderful day her father killed the pig he and a neighbor had raised together. Now they would have meat.

"For weeks we ate pork chops and head cheese and roast butt. Then a January thaw came, and there was no refrigeration for the carcass hanging in the back shed—and the thaw didn't last for a day, it lasted weeks.

"So Mother started her cooking marathon. She got jars, sealers, containers of every shape, and sterilized them. Then she fried the pork which Father had cut into narrow strips. She packed them into the jars, sealing them with grease. Four years later we were still eating that pork. At that time we lived in a three-room cottage (shack would have been a better name for it) and after her cooking marathon, we actually scraped the grease off the kitchen walls."

The Depression times weren't easy, but they molded character. "It was sink or swim together, so we pooled our resources and survived," said Mary. "There was no striving to keep up with the Joneses; we were the Joneses."

She recalled the fun times: "Our laughter broke the gloom. Neighbors would gather in someone's parlor, one of the men would bring a fiddle and the married couples would dance up a storm, while the children watched between the posts in the upstairs balustrade. We had sleigh-rides, skating parties and toboganning; they were fun things that didn't cost money."

However, holidays and special occasions often brought out the hurt and the loneliness, the bad as well as the good.

Sarah still remembers Easter 1933. "We hadn't seen an orange or a green since Christmas. About eight weeks before Easter Father started mysteriously disappearing every afternoon. We knew that in the morning, he made the rounds, looking for work.

"'You don't suppose father has—well—a friend?' my sister whispered to me when Father's away-from-home time became very noticeable.

"Of course I hotly denied such a supposition, but deep inside I wondered.

"On Easter morning Mother hid the eggs everyone had dipped and painted. Instead of Father participating as usual, he again disappeared.

"Two hours later, anyone could have cut the tension in the house with a knife. Then Father returned. Grinning broadly, he said, 'I have a present, something special for our Easter dinner.' He waved a bag in front of us.

"Mother was so angry she grabbed the bag out of his hand. Onto the table spilled lettuce, the leaves no bigger than a quarter, two dozen baby-finger-thin onions and some radishes the size of a dime.

"'Where—did you get all this?' Mother stammered, sitting on the nearest chair.

"Father's grin grew wider. 'Some weeks ago when you were saying we needed some greens in our diet, I got the idea of making a hot bed, but I didn't have any horse manure, and I didn't have the right spot to build on. I remembered Pete Reynolds had a horse stable in half of his L-shaped barn, and we needed something like that with a sheltered southern exposure, so I approached him. He liked the idea so much, he even helped me build the hot bed—and his family has lettuce and onions and radishes today too.'"

Sarah recalls that it wasn't the most churchly Easter morning, "but I believe we were all closer to God that morning than at any other time in our lives."

Sometimes, for those on the senior side, it is like living those moments over again to recall their youth. It was like this for Olivia, who lives in a nursing home. She loves to talk about when she was a young girl and the family lived on a small farm where her father market-gardened. "We certainly had plenty of food, but there weren't any luxuries. Even a small piece of chocolate was a treat."

Just the mention of chocolate brought back other memories, and she told how her parents had rented a couple of vacant upstairs rooms to a mother and her son who were on welfare. The mother, whose health had not been good, mainly because she hadn't been able to afford the proper food or medicine, suddenly caught pneumonia, and just a few days before Christmas, died.

Because it was difficult to find a place for the 12-year-old boy, Ross, he stayed on with Olivia's family. She recalled how Ross used to sit behind the old wood stove and play tunes like *The Red River Valley* on a comb covered with wax paper.

"Three days before Christmas, Mother and Dad had to deliver some potatoes in town, and Ross and I were left on our own. We decided to snoop; after all, we knew there was no Santa."

After about an hour of fruitless searching, the two found two chocolate Santas wrapped in celophane, tucked away at the back of the buffet.

"Mm, don't they look good," Olivia said.

Ross agreed. "You know, Livey, we could gnaw off the heads; that way your mother would just think the mice got into them."

On Christmas morning when the two rushed down to see what was under the tree, right out front were two headless—and middleless—Santas. Around the top of the boots, all that was left, was a note:

15

"Mother mouse likes chocolate too."

Ellie, who was 78, was sitting beside Olivia. She recalled one special Christmas, which usually was never much different from any other day at their house.

"There were just the three of us, Mother, Dad and me. We were never invited to any of the relatives, and we were too poor to invite them for a meal at our place."

That was the year her father had lost his hand in an accident. There wasn't any compensation to cover such things in the '30s. Her mother had told her that if she was a good girl, and since they didn't have a tree, maybe Santa would put a gift somewhere else for her—like on the windowsill.

That morning when she awoke, she tip-toed into the kitchen. There on the windowsill, in an unwrapped box, was the homeliest fountain pen and pencil set she had ever seen, yet, decades later, it was one of the "treasures" she brought to the nursing home with her.

Ellie was still able to recall her father's grace, as he blessed their Christmas dinner (stuffed cottontail, baked potatoes and preserved strawberries): "May those that have plenty be truly grateful—and those that have little, may they be comforted by the assurance of better days to come."

Rob, who had known both women in his youth, had been listening to Olivia's and Ellie's reminiscences.

"I remember one Christmas," he said, "there were seven of us and we lived in an upstairs apartment over a butcher shop. Mother used to scrub the meat counters and floors in payment for the rent; Dad picked up whatever job he could find."

After taking a couple of puffs on his pipe, Rob went on to say that a church group had left a box of

16

groceries and a pair of mittens for each of the children. He remembered someone had treated his Dad to a few drinks, and he had come home grumpy and miserable; that was when Rob and his older sister had decided to go for a walk. "We looked at all the beautiful trees in the windows; oh, how we envied those people!

"When we neared home, the man who owned the livery stable was just closing for the night; he sold Christmas trees as a sideline.

"'Why don't we ask him for those broken branches?' my sister said. 'Maybe we could bind them together and make a little tree.'"

And so Rob asked the liveryman if they might gather up some of the branches. "He stared at us for a long moment, then he told us to wait. In the corner of his yard was a pile of broken branches. Quickly he brushed them aside, and right at the bottom was a tree. Its trunk was twisted, its branches were crushed, but it was a tree and we dragged it home.

"Mother helped us put it in the living room while my brother filled an old bucket with coal for a stand. My youngest sister cut out a cardboard star and crayoned it yellow. My older sister made icicles from thin strips of foil from a pound of tea. We fashioned garlands from red wool and popcorn and draped the lower branches. Do you know, in all my years, I have never seen a more beautiful tree!"

Seniors in the '30s made the most out of everything they had, and their children learned to do the same. They created their own antics to relieve the boredom and the worry of no money, no work, and sometimes no hope. Everyone rolled with the punches.

There was one holiday 90-year-old Russell recalls. He and his brother had been to a fireworks display at the park. In those days firecrackers were not limited to sale only twenty-four hours before a holiday; they could be bought anytime, by anybody. Russell had a large firecracker still in his pocket, and he knew better than to go home with it—his father considered them "wastes of the devil."

"Why don't we throw it in the old well, the one at the side of the house?" his brother suggested.

Russell thought that was a good idea, but he had a better one: "Why don't we light it first?"

While Russell lighted the firecracker, his brother lifted the metal cover of the well. Then the two boys ran for the house.

They were about halfway up the stairs when an explosion rocked the house, and their father, scrambling into his pants, yelled "Fire! The house is on fire!"

Then he saw the boys, and somehow, just seeing them on the stairs, he knew they had something to do with the blast. Would you believe the boys ate their meals standing up for the next week?

Hallowe'en was always a good time for the young to let off some of their excess energies and have fun to boot. When Martin's grandson asked, "What did you do on Hallowe'en, Grandpa?" it was a time for him to reflect. Oh yes, the good old days—when streets were unpaved and the plumbing was outside—and grandmother made fudge and kids ducked for apples.

"Well, Grandpa," a gentle voice prodded from the other side of the room, "answer the boy. Tell him what you used to do!"

Martin chuckled a little. Well, when he was a boy his family lived just outside a small village, and there was a man in that village who ran the grist mill. "Never had a civil word for anyone."

One Hallowe'en a bunch of boys (Grandpa was about 14) decided to pay him for all his "kindnesses." They not only unloaded a wagon of feed he had left

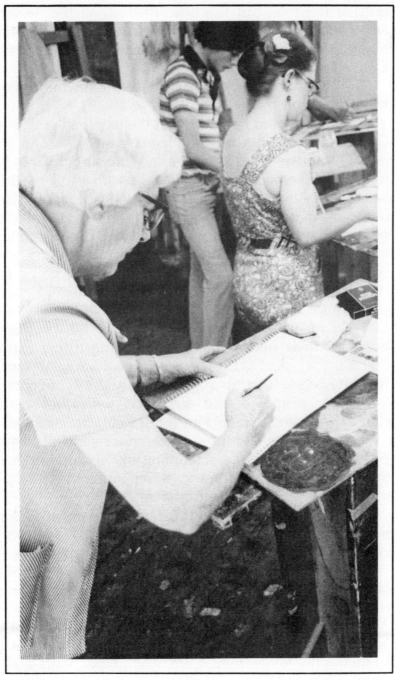

Lynda Middleton

outside the mill, but the boys dismantled the wagon and hauled every piece of it up onto the roof of the building where they put it back together again. They even reloaded the feed.

"You should have seen his face the next morning when he came to the mill!"

Grandpa didn't repeat what the man had said, but Grandma knew; her face reddened a bit.

Outhouses were always a favorite target, Grandpa recalled, especially their uncle's who lived on the next road. After the previous year, when he found his outhouse in his wife's prize nasturtium bed, the uncle vowed he was going to fix his nephews. He was going to weight down that outhouse until it was so heavy a block and tackle couldn't lift it, and he was going to rig it with several sets of sleigh bells. He would even the score.

By means of the local grapevine, the brothers heard of their uncle's plans, so, getting a few extra fellows, they decided to pay their visit early, in fact, just after dark (they usually visited about midnight).

"We struggled and struggled with that darn thing. We almost didn't move it," Martin laughed. "When we finally set it down, the door suddenly flew open and Aunt Hester, screaming like a banshee, her long skirts gathered high above her ankles, went leaping like a leprechaun to the house."

"That must have been a terrible experience for the poor woman," Grandma sympathized. "I understand she never again visited an outhouse after dark."

"Well, you didn't do so badly at those Hallowe'en parties you used to attend," her husband reminded her. "After all, that's where you met me."

"That was the night I touched those awful cat's eyes," Grandma shivered, remembering. "How was I supposed to know they were just grapes with their skins removed?"

"Wasn't that the party where poor Cousin Aimee actually thought she shook hands with a ghost and fainted dead away?"

Grandma giggled, "The ghost's hand being a glove you filled with oatmeal porridge."

For most seniors Hallowe'en is remembered as a fun time, a party time livened up with the antics of the exuberance of youth. These were the capers that lightened the dark days and made them human, but the stamp of the Depression left its imprint.

There was something else that left just as great an imprint, the workhouses, the poorhouses, the houses of refuge, where conditions were akin to those in the prisons. Inmates were segregated. A husband and wife committed to the same place could only meet clandestinely. Otherwise, they saw each other at chapel or on a rare night when someone brought entertainment.

The senile, the retarded, the slightly deranged and the old were all mixed together. Anyone who could work, worked. Most of the houses of refuge were more than partially self-supporting; they grew as much of their food as they could. While the men worked in the gardens and fields, the women performed household duties, cooking and preserving.

Morning breakfast was usually a bowl of mush (oatmeal porridge or cornmeal), a slice of bread and a cup of tea or hot water.

If a resident didn't cooperate or complained unduly, he or she was put into solitary confinement and fed bread and water.

The following are rules dealing with behaviour:

"Any person guilty of drunkenness, disobedience, immorality, obscenity, disorderly conduct, profane or indecorous language, theft, waste, or who shall absent himself or herself from the premises without the permission of the keeper, or who shall be guilty of injury or defacing any part of the home or furniture therein, or who shall commit waste of any kind, shall be punished as the case may seem to demand."

It wasn't just the residents of these houses of refuge who suffered, it was their families too. Can you imagine the horror of this rule?

"No visitor shall have admission to the home on the Sabbath Day without the consent of the keeper upon good cause shown."

Many of the so-called refuges were firetraps, and to make matters worse, all doors were kept locked—only the warden and matron had keys. Token health inspections were made regularly, and there was much ado about cleanliness. The residents, who were usually committed by a reeve or deputy, had to have a doctor's statement saying that the to-be-admitted indigent was free of communicable disease. These places didn't exist in some dark past, they existed until 1946 and in some areas even later.

The stigma of having one's relatives committed to the poor house clung to families for years. This dread of being institutionalized, even though now it means humane treatment and attractive surroundings, still tortures the minds and memories of seniors today.

The gentleness of the early 1900s, the War Years, the Roaring Twenties, the Great Depression and the catastrophic conditions of the poor houses, have all left an imprint on the lives of today's senior citizens. They want a better quality of life than their forefathers had, and they are using the signposts of the past to guide themselves into the future.

Changing Family and Social Relationships

Family and social relationships are changing, and for better or worse, seniors must change right along with them. The good old days are gone forever and our tomorrows are here. The quality of life we attain in the years to come will be greatly governed by our ability to change with the times.

Today's seniors are traveling a far different route than our forefathers did. They want to be family independent, not family dependent, although health does not always allow us to be master of our fate.

Parke Goodwin, 19th century American journalist, said, "Independence is the greatest of all human benefits, without which no other benefit can truly be enjoyed."

Seniors have the desire and the need to live on their own, separate from their children. Social Security and Old Age Security and its supplements have now provided them with the means to do that. This new-found financial freedom has allowed them the choice—they no longer have to accept a secondary role in someone else's house, they can chart their own lifestyle.

23

"When I can no longer live on my own, I have given my children specific instructions that they are to put me into an institution. I don't want to be a burden to anyone," one woman at a senior women's growth group said. Her feelings were echoed by many.

This woman had charted her course, but what about seniors who haven't made such a decision, who have left their lives in the hands of their children?

According to law, parents are responsible for minor children, but there are few laws stating that adult children are responsible for parents, and those only apply in special circumstances. In years past, a child in trouble was always welcome at his parents' home; adult children, then and now, do not always return the welcome.

There are some older citizens who bring enrichment and joy into an adult child's home. They are mature, not only in age, but also in understanding and tolerance. They are part of the family, yet wise enough to remain on the fringe to allow everyone breathing room with no need for artificial respiration.

Years ago it was not uncommon for four or five generations to live together—each had a particular role. Today, because these roles have lost their definition, even two generations have difficulty getting along in the same house. The aging parent's role has shifted.

Sometimes when a senior moves in with his or her family, the spouse moves out, leaving undreamed-of emotional repercussions and hard feelings. Families choose sides and one is pitted against the other, too often with the aging parent caught right in the middle.

Some of this changing of relationships, this shifting of roles, has been good. Women have entered the job market; now they are heads of families, and the servitude of running a multi-generation household under the tutelage of an aging mother or aunt has been trampled into oblivion.

The mobility of families has also had an effect on the changing roles of adult children and aging parents. Yet surveys show that six out of 10 adult children still live within driving distance of their parents, and in some areas this statistic is much higher.

Just what does a family in our materialistic society owe to an aging parent? Three things! *Respect:* The Bible teaches us we should honor our father and mother, but this respect must be earned throughout life—it is not a coat a senior can slip on with the passing years. *Love* is an emotion that can only be freely given; it can't be bought or demanded. *Duty* is an obligation, an undischarged debt that we owe to our families and ourselves, simply the "do as we would be done by" rule of thumb. But we do not owe a complete sacrifice of self!

The once-expected martyrdom of the youngest member of the family to the lifetime care of the aging parent has been swept into oblivion—martyrdom is demeaning to the parent and self-destructive to the child. There is no place in today's scheme of living for the whip-tongue of a domineering parent.

Sometimes roles must reverse themselves when a parent has to give up his or her independence because of illness or aging and become institutionalized. Often the adult child becomes the parent and the parent becomes the child. So that the parent's self-esteem is not cut to shreds, the reversal of roles should be treated more as a partnership, leaving the senior's dignity and self-respect, so much a part of the will to live, intact.

Some adult children take unfair advantage of this change in role relationship: they usurp their parents' decision-making rights and take over without a thought to their parents' feelings. They assume authority with the unyielding sternness of a regimental sergeant-major, and there are frequent confrontations between them and their seniors, who are afraid of the future and need encouragement and support. This tough, exacting approach does nothing to allay their fears or bring them comfort. When a parent must be institutionalized, there are three things to remember: don't overreact, don't overanticipate, don't overindulge. Just use good old TLC—Tender Loving Care!

Even in the realm of marriage, relationships are changing: people are parting after 30 and 40 years of supposedly wedded bliss. Other seniors are finding a richer, deeper meaning in marriage; for many, it is the first time that the two of them have been alone; there were always the children. Then, too, in their early years of marriage, before modern nursing homes and homes for the aged, the aging parent was an accepted part of their household. Now seniors are starting on a new relationship in which they only have to think of each other; it is a new marriage contract.

Some (luckily they are in the minority) are still searching for an elusive romantic love of their youth; these mythical loves were just that—mythical. True, in the past society put love aside for duty, but lost loves can't be recaptured.

When marriages fail, when a senior is widowed, some will search for a new partner. What are the chances of a senior having a successful marriage the second time around? Good, according to a marriage counsellor, providing—and "providing" is the catchword—they have thoroughly discussed their plans with both her family and his family by previous marriage.

It isn't that the families are against a marriage, they are against the changing of inheritance rights.

More second marriages are wrecked by family quarrels than for any other reason. Seniors just can't discard their families, they are a part of their lives. Even in a second marriage they still need their family's understanding and loyalty.

By the time most seniors contemplate a second marriage, they have accumulated a house, savings bonds, a car, maybe a retirement fund, and quite often there has been insurance money claimed for the death of a spouse. Generally, they are better off financially than when they went into their first marriage.

Money is too often the problem between husband and wife in an October-November relationship. Before marriage is seriously considered, seniors should plan out what assets belong to his side, what assets belong to her side, and what assets belong to both of them. This should be written down in their wills.

In the changing relationships between men and women over the years, sex is often a problem. It can be a problem in a first-time-around relationship as well as in a second-time-around situation. Sex is not something reserved only for the young, it can be enjoyed by all ages.

One of the main causes of sexual inadequacy is the absence of sexual activity. A widow or widower does not have the opportunity once available for sexual intimacy. If a widower marries a year or so after the death of his wife, he will often experience difficulty, even though in a study made at the Duke University Center, it was verified that "persons who were sexually active during youth and middle age are more likely to retain that same activity in old age."

Some women, once they are free of childbearing or past menopause, find sex repugnant. This is not due to age, but to attitude. Sexual incapacity is rooted to cultural rather than biological standards—sex is associated with the younger woman, not the older. A man can find someone to have sex with for money, but for a woman there isn't the same opportunity.

Gerontologists tell us that seniors have been sexually brainwashed. It is true the sexual response may be slowed by the aging process, but it certainly doesn't disappear.

Many seniors, especially women, turn away from a second marriage because of the sex aspect. The body changes as we grow older; in a woman the vagina becomes shorter and narrower, and is less elastic. In men, an erection can take longer, bringing on anxieties about sexual performance. Worrying about impotence can make one impotent.

Experimental studies have shown that on the average, married couples in their sixties and seventies have sex from twice a week to at least once a month. Although age has slowed them, their pleasures have not diminished.

Sex has come out of the closet for the young and middle aged; now it is time it came out for grandma and grandpa. If two people share love or companionship, there is no reason why they can't share a sexual relationship.

Married couples in nursing homes suffer the most—they simply have no privacy. Sex is not a dangerous activity for seniors; it is one that can release tension and frustration as well as bringing meaning into life.

Sex education and marital counseling, according to some gerontologists, are becoming as important in the later years as they were in youth. Breakdown of marriage can happen at any age, and often sex is partly to blame.

Seniors have to change with the times. They have to put the biases of the past where they belong, in the past. They have to reach out for new relationships to replace ones that have been lost; if a second marriage is the answer, then why not? Second marriages are not just an extension of the first; they are a new and separate entity.

In years past, marriage was the only acceptable pursuit for women; they married because it was expected of them. Now with the liberation of their daughters and granddaughters, many grandmothers are finding in their widowhood the freedom they desired, and are reveling in it.

Others are moving into common-law relationships, some by choice, others by necessity. Although still frowned on by many, these relationships are being recognized by social workers, and are even being incorporated into application forms for pensions, making a common-law partner eligible for spouse's benefits after a certain length of time.

The needs of seniors go deeper than accepted social standards. For instance, when a senior had a spouse in a nursing home, and divorce is not an acceptable solution, his or her needs and desires still need fulfilment. When he or she finds someone to share life with, they enter into a common-law relationship. And who should judge?

These are our times, and people are more important than the rigid rules of the past.

The Road to Retirement and Beyond

Retirement means finding a new way of life, and despite all that seniors have heard and read about how wonderful it is, retirement isn't Utopia. We have been educated to work; now we must be educated to retire.

So that the quality of our lives can be maintained during these later years, we need clear signposts, we need direction and purpose. Retirement isn't intended to be a form of suspended animation; it is a time to get involved and to do the things we want to do—a time to enjoy the fruits of our labors.

For some, retirement is a nightmare from which there is, in their opinion, only one escape. Unfortunately the suicide rate is as high in the older age brackets as it is among the young. It is a paradox that people spend a third of their lives preparing for their jobs, another third working at them, and yet they leave the rest of their lives to chance—chance rarely pays off.

The main purpose of pre-retirement workshops, seminars and night courses is to make those who are approaching the senior side more aware of the options and alternatives that are available to them.

Although two and a half million Canadians are already over 65 years of age, most are certainly not ready for the rocking chair. They are youthful, energetic and knowledgeable, with expertise in every area of life, and they want more than to be just a statistic in our society.

Jack L. Lerette, former president of the National Pensioners and Senior Citizens Federation, says, "From my experience, I can say that the ones who make some preparation before they retire are the happiest."

Pre-retirement seminars and workshops can bring knowledgeable speakers in geriatrics, finance, health and leisure to groups of seniors who otherwise would not have the opportunity of hearing them. To varying extents, everyone has some fear of growing old, so proper counselling is as important at this stage as it was when we were young and needed guidance about the future. Also, we need to understand the changing process of our bodies so that the positive aspects of retirement can be developed to the fullest extent.

Most people who are involved in pre-retirement courses believe that if a senior hasn't started planning for retirement before he or she reaches 55, it is already too late. One person who disagrees with this theory is Myrtle Brodsky who began her writing career at age 80. Now, seven years later, she is sought after as a speaker on "how it feels to be 87." Her writing, which often describes travelling by bus (she has no car), is read with great interest by seniors and other age groups who prefer to travel by motor coach.

"My life just went from one stage to the other without any conscious effort on my part," she says. Her life is proof of her belief that our bodies adjust themselves to these slower-paced years. If we accept the aging process and work with it instead of against it,

31

we will pass into retirement without trauma, an adjustment that may be easier for housewives than for those men coming directly from the workforce.

At a recent pre-retirement seminar, one man recalled, "It was like dropping into an abyss. There was nothing! It took me two years to get my bearings—two years before I had any desire to get up in the morning."

Since the brain is the motor of the body, we have to be mentally as well as physically active. Up to now, time has employed us; now we must employ time. In retirement a senior will have approximately 2,000 extra hours per year to do exactly what he or she wants to do. Up to now we have been the "taking" generation; now we should become part of the "giving" generation."

Gerontologist Sister St. Michael Guinan has said, "By wasting our time, our energies, the potentials God gave us, we are robbing future generations of a wealth of knowledge and expertise."

One man who certainly hasn't robbed the world of his expertise is Dr. Albert E. Berry, retired general manager and chief engineer of the Ontario Water Resources Commission. Judging from his schedule, it's hard to believe that he is retired.

In September 1978, well past his 80th birthday, he was in Chicago where he was the first Canadian to receive an honorary membership in the American Public Works Association. A few weeks later he attended a conference of the Water Pollution Control Federation in Philadelphia.

Berry, who earned his doctorate at the University of Toronto, was guest speaker at his alma mater's sesquicentennial celebration. Between his speaking engagements he is drafting a book and enjoying more than a dozen crafts in which he excels—all this, and he is past 80. "I didn't really retire," he says. "I just changed jobs."

Since leaving his post in 1963, he has been acting as a consultant for the Conservation Council of Ontario. He also acts as consultant for the United Nations' World Health Organization, which sends him all over the globe. WHO first offered him the job about 11 years ago, but at that time his wife was chronically ill and he could not accept. Later, he wrote WHO saying he was free to travel. "I didn't hear from them for several months, then one day I got a letter asking me to go to Bangkok, Thailand."

In Bangkok, Berry was to join a retired German engineer who was also an expert in the water and sewage field. The two men were asked to study a sewer system proposal by a firm of U.S. consulting engineers. Since the project was to be funded by the World Bank, that body wanted the approval of WHO before providing the money.

"It was a very interesting few months," Berry says. He and his associate travelled by foot and by boat over Bangkok's 10 kilometers of canals, or klongs as they are called in Thai.

Since the only sewers in the city are storm sewers, the klongs carry all the waste to the Chao Phraya River that flows into the Gulf of Siam. The U.S. firm proposed a sewage plant at the edge of the city. Berry and his associate felt it should be built near the mouth of the river, located 10 miles farther downstream. Reluctantly the firm changed its design to meet the consultants' recommendations.

"It was remarkable how well my associate and I worked together. We were of different nationalities, different backgrounds, yet we agreed on every point," Dr. Berry says. The German engineer spoke English, but had difficulty writing it, so the Canadian consultant did the paperwork.

When this man left Bangkok, the government presented him with a cigarette case, which he treasures, although he has many mementoes from all over the world.

At home his interest turns to less adventurous pursuits like craftwork. "Seniors can do a lot of things if they really want to do them," he says.

In the hobby room in his basement he has chairs he has re-upholstered, others he has refinished, some he has caned. "Caning is becoming a lost art," he adds, "but it can be mastered."

Dr. Berry is also an accomplished painter and photographer and his wood carving can be seen on the hymnal board at a local church. Leathercraft and leather tooling are also among his crafts.

For many, retirement is the end of the road. For this man, it is just another dimension of an active life.

Howard, on the other hand, is a different type of person; he finds "just existing" enough. He doesn't choose to live beyond the frame of his own little world.

For 28 years he was an insurance agent; his sales were good and he made a lot of money. Then he had a heart attack and it frightened him. Although the doctor, after his recovery, advised him to slow down a bit, Howard took an early retirement.

Now he gets up about nine each morning, showers and shaves, goes down to the local doughnut shop for coffee and a muffin, and for the next hour-and-a-half, talks to friends and acquaintances. At about eleven, he picks up the morning paper and goes home; reads it until lunch, then watches the afternoon movie. Depending on the weather and the time of year, he'll either cut the lawn or shovel a little snow; sometimes he will even consent to go shopping with his wife. After dinner the couple usually play bridge, attend a concert or watch TV.

In all appearances Howard is experiencing a successful retirement. He literally drifts from one day to the next without challenges, without any highs or lows. For him, drifting is enough—and there are many Howards across North America; an easy, unruffled lifestyle is all they desire.

For Arnold, a retired mechanic, this isn't enough. For the first few months he enjoyed his freedom. Then, suddenly, he became tired. The longer he was retired, the more fatigued he became. In fact, he didn't even want to get out of bed for breakfast—he asked his wife to bring it to him. He was 66, yet he felt old mentally and physically. He believed there was nothing ahead for him but the grave, and subconsciously he was just lying down to die.

Dr. Hans Selye, noted expert on stress and aging, has said, "Just as our muscles become flabby and degenerate, so will our brain if we don't use it for something useful; it will slip into chaos and confusion."

And this was what was happening to Arnold. He found his work meaningful; without it, life had no purpose, no quality—he was lost. Jack L. Lerette confirms that seniors who don't use their minds and their physical capabilities when they retire, deteriorate faster than those who have interest. "I have seen people just disintegrate and die within three years."

Retirement isn't only a matter of money or travel; it also has a great deal to do with friends. For many, friendships have been built through the work sphere; when we no longer work, this sphere is going to grow considerably smaller—it can even vanish. It's essential to build interests away from work because new interests usually bring new friends and acquaintances. If there was only a work sphere before retirement, it won't be easy, but then who said growing old was easy?

Women, too, are affected by the retirement process. Although the wife, in many cases, has been absent from the workforce, her lifestyle is going to change when her mate retires. When the breadwinner no longer goes to work, she is going to find a good many of her independent activities have to be cancelled; her leisure hours will now be aligned with those of her spouse.

Martin was a cook in one of the better restaurants. When he retired, he said, "I never want to look at food again." After a month's vacation, Martin was ready to go back to work, only now there was no work to go back to. He invaded his wife's kitchen; she couldn't even boil water properly.

In desperation, she got him working on recipes for one or two people. He made changes; he tested recipes; and together they put together a booklet. Then, because of money problems, they moved to a resort area where they live in a house rent-free and he works as a cook during the summer. In the winter they will be working on another booklet.

When a husband retires, often it seems that the wife just goes along for the ride. That's what happened to Connie. "When I retire we're going to move to our cottage," Jim said. Both spent many hours fixing up the place until it was just the way they wanted it. Then winter came and Jim went hunting and ice fishing and took part in all the winter activities. Connie was left alone in the cabin; she was cut off from her friends and the companionship of her weekly quilting club. She became morose and depressed; her body just didn't want to function properly.

Next came the storm, and they were isolated for

weeks. Connie sank deeper into depression and finally an ambulance crew brought her out on a snowmobile sled.

Her basic problems were boredom, frustration and isolation. The Utopian cabin was fine for Jim, but it was a destructive environment for Connie. In the winter she had nothing to do with her time and it almost destroyed her.

Mel and Ida had a different problem. For 28 years he earned his living at a job he hated; he could hardly wait to see the last of the knitting mill where he worked as a weaver. With a large family to support, he had stuck it out to the bitter end. Now he wanted to travel.

Ida went along with the idea; they bought a camper, painted it and fixed it up until it became a dream home inside. There was only one hitch. After their oldest girl had married, Ida had gone back to work as a legal secretary. She loved her job and she didn't want to give it up.

"Why can't we just travel for a month?" she asked Mel. The firm she worked for said they would grant her an extra two or three weeks vacation time.

That wasn't good enough for Mel. He wanted to go on a cross-country trip. When he finished that he wanted to go to Florida for four or five months. In the summertime, he wanted to fish at a little lake in the woods.

"What about my job?" Ida protested. "And our home?"

"We're going to sell," he answered, and sell they did. The money was put into a high-interest savings account, and he and Ida moved into an apartment temporarily. "As far as your job is concerned," he said, "you can just quit."

There was no way Ida could see herself frittering

away the endless hours, vacationing 52 weeks of the year. She was an energetic, vibrant person who needed her family and people around her. Mel and Ida separated—their ways of life were no longer reconcilable.

Retirement can be devastating to a couple whose marriage has only been just tolerable. Both still need interests apart from each other so that their time together will be limited. Yet other couples have found their lives have never been happier. Innis and Mae lived on a farm. When he became ill, they sold it and moved to a ranch style house in the suburbs. At first Innis found the hours hard to fill. One day Mae admonished him: "You know you could refinish that chair of my mother's. I have been asking you to do it for years—and you always said you didn't have time. Well . . . ."

Innis refinished the chair; it was beautiful. When his daughter-in-law saw it, she asked him to refinish a chest of drawers for the grandson's room. That was the beginning. Innis loves refinishing—making things beautiful again. He is under no pressure: he works when he feels like it. In his basement workshop, he is apart from Mae, although it is surprising how often she sneaks down with a cup of tea.

Mae's hours are filled with keeping house, knitting and crocheting, and making the best strawberry jam in the country.

"We have never been happier in our lives," Innis confirmed, reaching for his wife's hand.

It is not necessary in retirement to follow one's former job pattern. For some seniors, especially those who now have single status, it is time to follow that youthful dream.

Audrey lost her husband the same month she retired from being a cashier at a local supermarket.

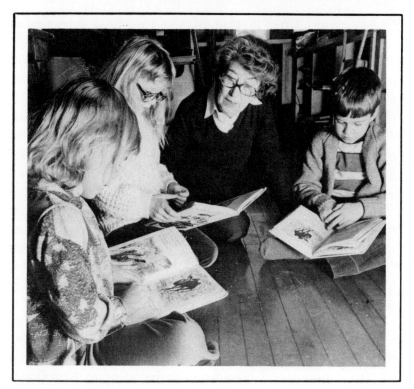

Rick Eglinton/The London Free Press

The couple had planned to travel, but she had no desire to go on her own. She had always wanted to be a librarian; she took some night courses and now she is a volunteer at a local nursing home where disabled people need the stimulus of books.

One 90 year old presented her with a great challenge. He liked books, but for his level of education, they were too long and often too deep, and he lost interest. Audrey found the solution in the children's library. "Now that his reading appetite is piqued, we just can't keep him supplied with books," she says. Even though this man can't walk, he is alert and happy, and Audrey is fulfiling an old dream.

Wasted time is one of the foremost enemies of retirement. Sid was a truck driver; for 47 years trucking had been his life. Upon retirement, he didn't know how to fill the hours. Finally, he answered a radio call for volunteers. Now Sid is a part-time volunteer for the cancer society; he drives patients to and from the cancer clinic. Although his expenses are paid, he receives no pay for his time. "It doesn't matter: at least I am useful again," he says.

Molly had a Masters degree in Group Work Therapy. After graduation she had lived in a settlement house in Chicago, where someone gave her an unwanted dog. When a friend started an obedience class for "mutts," she asked Molly to bring her dog along. Molly went "just for kicks," but an interest in animal training was sparked by the experience.

Now, at age 64, Molly is retired. "When I left nursing, I had to find something to do or go crazy. And then in the supermarket one day I heard someone mention he would like to take his dog to obedience classes, but there were none in the area. That gave me the idea."

Besides teaching dog obedience, Molly travels to seminars and workshops throughout Canada and the United States, learning new obedience patterns and techniques. Although she has a few health problems, she is happy and well-adjusted; her life has meaning.

Retirement isn't the end of the road. It is a time to begin again, a period to create, to participate, to find new areas of personal achievement, to make new friends and to serve others. It is a time to live, not just exist!

Leisure

Leisure is like a beautiful garment; it cannot stand constant wear. When we reach retirement, we are going to have at least 2,000 extra hours of leisure per year. If we are going to receive any benefit from all these extra hours, they must, like work, give us something in return.

Leisure should give us three things: a sense of accomplishment; a sense of worth as human beings; a sense of pleasure. No matter what path we follow—a third career, volunteerism, hobbies, crafts, travel or education—we must receive one or more of these three fulfilments if life is going to be rich and rewarding.

If we have been wise, we already have an outside interest or hobby. If we haven't, and retirement is just around the corner, then those 2,000 hours are going to seem endless. Often you hear seniors say, "At my age, I just can't try something new!" Why not?

Winston Churchill came to power a few months after he had reached his 65th birthday, and what would the world have done without him? Six years after today's mandatory retirement age, Michelangelo not only designed the dome of St. Peter's in Rome, he undertook to complete the cathedral's construction.

Don't let your conception or society's conception of age put you out to pasture. You *can* develop new interests, have a third career and contribute to the quality of life.

Some seniors are using their talents abroad through international volunteer agencies. These volunteers receive only expense money, but their work is meaningful; they are upgrading their own sense of worth, and they are accomplishing something worthwhile.

After 40 years in the pulp and paper industry, George Wilson and his wife Fran went to Korea to work with Koreans developing their pulp and paper industry. "It helps keep you young, although it's not very comfortable living," George said. He and Fran also spent two months in India in 1975.

There's an old saying: "You can't teach an old dog new tricks." We know that isn't true. Since no one has told the dog he's old, he just goes right on learning. Seniors, too, are going right on with their learning: they're going back to school, to colleges, to universities, and taking night courses, as well as earning daytime credits, and governments are waiving part of the cost. At one college, more than 1,500 credit courses and 29 academic departments are available to seniors.

There is a lesson for all of us to learn in the example set by Helen Richards Campbell who at 81 received her Bachelor of Arts degree, the oldest person ever to graduate from her university.

Seniors don't have to be academically-minded to go back to school. There are many subjects they can take just for the pleasure of learning: current events, yoga, creative writing, painting and the art of designing and creating craftwork. Often in these courses it is a senior who is doing the teaching.

A real hobby is not just a way to kill time, it is an occupation that lets you do something creative in a useful way, and the choices for being creative are as vast and wonderful as our minds will let them be.

Some seniors are restoring old furniture; others are giving new life to old crafts such as caning and bookbinding. One man with a small acreage took up goatherding, supplementing his income by selling the meat and milk, which is especially good for those who have trouble digesting cow's milk. Another chap, whose hobby was bees, went into it as a full-time business.

Len is a retired movie theatre projectionist. He is also a ham radio operator and from his comfortable living room he can talk to people all over Canada and the United States. When the F2 layer is right, his transmissions go even farther afield.

Through his membership in the Radio Society, he heard of a project to help the blind "to get them away from the four walls of their apartments by means of sound."

Len wrote to the Canadian National Institute for the Blind and offered his services. He didn't hear a thing from them; then, four years later, a letter came, there was a need in his area. They needed a sighted person to instruct, coach and encourage a whitecaner. Len was excited; this was the challenge he had been waiting for. Even for a person with full vision it takes hours of study and concentration; for the handicapped, the hours are multiplied tenfold.

Eleven months later, when his ham trainee received her license, Len was on cloud nine: "I was just as thrilled as the day I received my own license."

Now he has two more whitecaners interested in becoming ham radio operators. Through sound, the four walls that often imprison them will be broken down. "It is one of the most rewarding undertakings of my life," he says.

Alta Cox wanted to play the piano. Her children received lessons, but she was never able to realize her ambition until she was 72. "It was now or never," she says with a laugh, flexing her arthritic fingers, which have improved greatly through her musical exercise.

Activity keeps us young. Our I.Q. does not decline with age; in fact, according to a recent study by the National Institute of Mental Health, judgment improves with the years.

Martha Gray was in a nursing home, and through its activity program was able to develop her talent for painting, and now sells many canvases to local people. When her eyesight failed, she turned to sculpting. "Now I see with my hands," she says, and another world has opened up to her.

Merv worked in a plywood factory office, and every few months samples of all the beautiful plywoods of the world came across his desk. "They were too nice to throw away, so I kept them, taking them home and stockpiling them in my basement workshop." After he retired, he became bored. Always interested in design, one rainy afternoon he decided to do something with his plywood. Now he is making trays fashioned from all the woods of the world, inlaid with stars and flowers. He has a lucrative hobby (people are waiting for their specially designed pieces), and he has a sense of worth as a human being. Merv has been confined to a wheelchair for the last twelve years.

It's true that seniors need plenty of time to rest, but they need opportunity too—opportunity to be somebodies instead of nobodies; like Merv, they need productive leisure.

There are hundreds of seniors who can't write, paint, hook a rug, or fire a ceramic, but they are excellent organizers. They get their sense of accomplishment through the achievements of others.

Woodbury is a small community, like a thousand others. They have a village drop-in centre which is used twice a month for bridge or a pot-luck supper. And they had one other resource—they had Verne. When she retired at age 69 from her job as salesperson specializing in china at a local gift store, she was bored, unhappy and frustrated; the hours loomed ahead endlessly. Then someone mentioned that the community needed a writers' group; she organized it, and now several of its members are being published. She organized a dilettante club for artists, then a current events discussion group to which political speakers are invited. Through her efforts, the senior community in Woodbury came alive.

Only a few seniors are content to spend all their leisure time playing bridge or euchre; most want a deeper form of expression than the pleasurable sociability of cards. This expression often needs money, and project money is not always easy to come by.

In 1972, the Canadian government launched its New Horizons program. The Federal Department of Health and Welfare developed this new program primarily to help reduce the sense of loneliness, isolation and inactivity that older people experience by giving them a chance to choose and develop projects that use their skills and talents, or pique their interest. The accent is on local needs, and each project must qualify on its own merit.

To be eligible, a group must consist of ten or more senior volunteers and the direction and management of the proposed activity must be in their hands. These grants can be used for recreation, fitness, education, to promote discussion, or for social services. New Horizons has funded everything from musical groups who entertain at nursing homes and homes for the aged to an airplane that never did get off the drawing board, and even pots and pans and kitchen sinks for drop-in centres.

New Horizons considers its grants as "seed funding," usually a one-shot boost to get a project in motion. After a specific time, about 18 months, the project must stand on its own feet and be self-supporting. Although most projects cost under $10,000, there's a ceiling of $100,000. Organizers must keep accurate financial records that are subject to audit by New Horizons; to date over 8,000 projects have been funded across Canada.

Yet with all this potential for useful activity made available, a good many seniors still sit at home, lonely and alone. Records show less than 35%, and in some areas less than 10%, take advantage of community-sponsored programs at churches, drop-in centers or organized recreational facilities.

Some prefer "to do their own thing" and this is one of the reasons travel, especially travel by bus, has vaulted to the fore in using up a goodly portion of those 2,000 extra hours in our retirement lives. By charter bus for minimal cost a senior can journey across Canada and the United States. True, you share a room unless you want to pay extra, but in terms of saving money, this mode of travel can't be beaten.

Seniors who can't afford to travel abroad or who don't for health reasons are taking short charter jaunts for a day or overnight, visiting museums, art shows, live theatre, botanical gardens and musical events, baseball and hockey games, all within their immediate area.

Many hotels and motels are offering 10% discounts to seniors, but these discounts are not usually available if booked through a travel agent.

In 1978 a group of veterans from both world wars, patients at a veterans' hospital, with the help of their activity director William Powell, chartered a plane and took a trip to Florida. Many of these men and women hadn't been outside the confines of the hospital in 20 years or more. By taking lessons, in such things as how to eat in a restaurant and how to cope in crowds, with the assistance of the coordinator, a nurse and two orderlies, they were able to function successfully.

Because of cost, seniors in increasing numbers are taking to the highways in vans, campers and tent trailers, and parks are offering camp sites at reasonable costs. Some adventurous oldsters are venturing deep into the north country; others are keeping to the more-developed recreational and conservation areas.

Regardless of how you spend your extra 2,000 hours of leisure, make sure the hours are productive, that they bring a sense of accomplishment, a sense of worth and a sense of pleasure. Whatever your way, fill your hours to the brim—they won't come this way again.

Spiritual, Mental and Physical Well-Being

"The health of our mind is of far more consequence to happiness than the health of our body." This statement was made in the early 19th century by clergyman Caleb Colton, and it's just as true today as it was then.

Our health and our spiritual well-being go hand in hand. Health is the ship on which we travel through life, and our faith is the compass we use to chart our course. When the health of the mind deteriorates, we get into all sorts of dark waters like depression and suicide, often the result of an irreversible progression of losses which can leave a senior's life without a sense of direction or purpose.

The mind rules the body, and when it loses its sense of direction, we flounder, unless we have the support of family and friends to help guide us to safe harbor. Unfortunately, many don't want to be bothered—they're too busy or too far away—and we can feel that no one really cares.

The worries of the aged are increasing instead of

decreasing. In the United States almost 25% of the total number of suicides are seniors, yet seniors make up only 10% of the population.

What have older persons got to worry about? They have their pension and a place to live—what else do they need? It's true that money and shelter are important, but it is the quality, not the security of their lives that seniors question. They are old; they are lonely; their memories are fading; pain racks their bodies; self-disdain has replaced self-esteem. For them, their worth as human beings seems gone.

In Japan, where 75% of families still follow the centuries-old custom of living with their oldest son, many of their "graying" population is "going to the mountains." Soji Tanaka, a specialist on the elderly in Japan's health and welfare ministry, says, "It's like an old Japanese fable. When a parent feels he or she has become a burden to their children, they ask to be taken to the mountains to die." The mountain for many of Japan's graying population is suicide.

This progressive, highly industrialized country has the second highest rate of suicide among the elderly in the world. Why? The reasons are many, although gerontologists point out that most companies retire their employees at 55; government pensions don't begin until 65, and more and more parents, because of cramped apartments, are forced to live alone or to go to nursing homes or special experimental old age communities. Some seniors just can't make the compromise between the traditions of the past with the progress of the present. It is a struggle that is just beginning—by the year 2015, Japan expects to have 25% of their population on the senior side.

Yet in other parts of the world where climate is harsh, life is austere and lonely, and poverty and unemployment are no strangers to the people, the suicide rate is low. Researchers believe it has something to do with people's religious faith, their strong ties to basic values, their inherent respect for the aged.

Canadian political leader Robert Stanfield, himself a senior citizen, says, "A policy of continuing activity for the aging is a challenge for enterprise, a challenge for government."

In their younger years, seniors' lives were motivated by challenge, both mental and spiritual. Their lives had an influence on others, their ideas were seriously considered, their actions had meaning. Now they need challenge and motivation on an individual level. We must exist for a reason—a reason we can believe in and accept.

Although suicide is widely discussed as a problem among our young, senior suicide goes unmentioned and unreported. Dr. Allen Willner, a psychologist who directs the Senior Citizen Treatment Program at Long Island Jewish-Hillside Medical Center, says, "For every reported suicide, there is one that is not reported."

There are many ways older persons can take their own lives without putting a gun to the head. Seniors fail to take medication or take too much (an "accidental" overdose), quit eating or have a car accident or pedestrian accident. Just stepping off the curb into traffic at the wrong moment is all that it takes.

Why do these suicides go unreported? Mainly, gerontologists believe, because death for an old person is an expected event, and consequently is less likely to be questioned. Also, the treatment of depression associated with suicide in our older population is complicated by the side-effects of many anti-depressant drugs, which react differently in older bodies.

But before we begin the treatment, we must attack the cause. We must put challenge and motivation back into lives which have become mundane, lives that are filled with guilt and regret for what might have been.

"A healthy spiritual outlook is the best preventive medicine we have," says Chaplain Charles Scott, a pastoral counselor and consultant. He believes health and religion are interrelated. "Unless we have inner peace, unless we come to terms with our guilts and fears, our health is going to suffer."

Scott is just one of 28 ministers of all faiths hired by the Ontario government to work in therapeutic ministry. Although he has been working as a community chaplain for 16 years, the last 11 have been devoted to those on the senior side of their lives.

Guilt is deep-rooted in many of our elderly because "not talking about problems, keeping grief locked inside, not letting others know we are hurting" is our heritage from the past.

Chaplain Scott has his own special way of helping seniors come to grips with their problems: "I usually ask—what does spirituality mean to you? Since people are all different, so is their concept of spirituality. More important, though, is the fact they are talking about religion, what they believe in, how they see it."

After this, Scott encourages seniors to talk about their own journey through life, their own personal ups and downs—where are they going, and how do they see the aging process?

One of the biggest stumbling blocks in coming to grips with life is memory, and Charles Scott puts special emphasis on "the healing of memories." Memories need to be talked about—not just the good ones, but the bad ones too. They have to be brought out into the open, examined and put into their proper perspective. "There is no use worrying about what you did or should have done in 1910. It is what you are doing now that is important." Shakespeare put it more bluntly: "What is done, is done!"

"The need of love" is very much a part of this chaplain's therapeutic ministry. "We all need love," he says, "and seniors more than most." This need is tied to the will to live. Unless an elderly person has someone who cares, life is meaningless and depression becomes the forerunner of other ills.

Seniors need something constant to hang onto; in the past, religion has been that constant, now in the light of new doctrines, even the faith of our fathers has been twisted into an unrecognizable shape. For older people, religion is the last rock on which they can firmly stand, and with the rushing currents of time eroding this foundation, they are fearful; the quality of life they foresaw for themselves has been washed away.

Now, in the face of this change, seniors must search for new challenges, new motivations to give their later years purpose and meaning. Only with a healthy mental and spiritual attitude can we bring quality to this senior side of living.

Nutrition

The motto for those on the senior side, as far as nutrition is concerned, should be: Eat Well To Feel Well. While proper diet is not going to cure all the ills of aging, it is going to postpone and possibly remove altogether some of the problems.

For some, nutrition means a too-good-eating way of living; unfortunately for others it is an unappetizing habit of tea and toast. Over 65% of the senior population has a nutritional deficiency. These men and women are not undernourished because they do not have enough to eat, they are undernourished because they do not eat the right kinds of foods.

Although our need for calories may decrease as we grow older (depending on how active we are—a man at 70 needs about 2000 calories and a woman about 1500), our need for vitamins, minerals, protein and other nutrients remains the same. There are approximately 57 nutrients or chemical compounds obtained from food used by the human body. The trick, of course, is to rebalance our diet.

There are four categories of food that should be

eaten each day to maintain good health:
    milk and milk products
    meat and alternatives
    fruits and vegetables
    bread and cereals

Each group has its own job to do. When we neglect eating vegetables or fruits or any of the other categories, we are simply short-changing our bodies.

Dr. Jean Mayer of Harvard, who has studied the nutritional problems of seniors says, "Many people when they see older persons begin to fail, assume they are just growing old. I've observed many seemingly senile patients admitted to a hospital who, after a few days on a hospital diet, became alert and rational."

While it's true senior citizens need less of the energy foods, they do need as much of the repair materials in food as they did at age 30. Our bodies need calcium, found in milk and milk products, to build and maintain good teeth and strong bones. Fruits, often called our protective foods, supply us with a wide variety of vitamins and minerals. Vegetables, too, give us necessary protection against disease. Enriched breads and wholegrain cereals not only give bulk to our diets, but also supply us with necessary vitamins. Meat and fish give us protein to repair worn-out tissue.

But most seniors require more fiber in their diets. Fiber is found in fruits, vegetables, wholegrain breads and cereals. Wheat bran is especially high in fiber content. Actually, fiber is a part of the plant material that we cannot digest, and since it is not digested, dietary fiber is not a source of energy or nutrients, but it is essential to health. It's a good regulator.

Diets low in fiber are sometimes referred to as "diseases of civilization." Dr. Denis Burkitt, a surgeon who spent 18 years in Africa, believes our food is lacking in something, and that something is fiber. Africans who have high-fiber diets do not suffer from heart disease, cancer of the bowel or obesity. "North Americans spend $250 million a year alone on laxatives. We could save ourselves a lot of discomfort and money by putting fiber back in our diets."

What does fiber do? It remains in the intestines as a bulky mass that helps remove the wastes left after the foods are digested and absorbed. Like a sponge, fiber takes in large amounts of water; stools are softer, bulkier and heavier. This stretches the intestinal wall which in turn helps promote regularity and muscle tone.

Over the years our taste buds have changed; now our appetites need to be re-educated. Sometimes medication will alter their sensitivity; for others, special diets restrict the variety of foods. The same foods eaten day after day can become dull, monotonous and destructive to appetite. This is where seniors need to put the ingenuity of their years to work. Besides, now they have plenty of time to experiment with foods.

For breakfast, why not try a soft-boiled egg in a fancy cup, and a sliced banana served in orange juice, with an English muffin smothered with your favorite marmalade, jam or honey?

If you have a problem with bread going stale before you've finished the loaf, why not try making French toast with orange juice added to the egg mixture? Salmon, too, can be served in a variety of ways. Instead of slamming two slices of bread together and bisecting it, cut your sandwich into four and garnish with a pickle, all served on a fancy plate. What if these are your good dishes—don't you want to enjoy them?

But, some seniors say, it's the cost! The price of food has skyrocketed. By choosing foods that are less expensive, yet contain the same nutritional value, health need not be impaired by a small budget.

Chicken wings are still fairly economical. Cover them with a sauce made from a little prepared mustard, Worcestershire sauce, butter, salt and lemon juice, and bake them with a potato that can be dressed up by serving with a little cheese, onion greens or parsley.

Seniors can use buttermilk instead of commercial yogurt, apples instead of avocados, tuna instead of salmon, oatmeal instead of sugar-coated cereals, and still retain nutritional value.

If someone has trouble cutting or otherwise handling their food, why not prepare meat in strips and leave off the gravy? It is tasty and can be eaten with the fingers; also, meat wrapped in a pastry or biscuit dough is "finger-lickin' good."

There are people in this older generation who say they can't cook a good meal because they have only a hot plate or a two-burner stove in their rooms, and only limited refrigeration. There's no doubt this can be a handicap, but there are ways to cope. A good skillet and a double or triple boiler will suffice for cooking; as for choice of foods, why not purchase items that don't need refrigeration? There are instant soups and instant cereals and plenty of variety in canned goods.

After extensive research, the Senate Select Committee on Nutrition and Human Needs has released its report on dietary goals, which states that simple procedures could improve everyone's health. They suggest we start by cutting down on salt and sugar. The report advises cutting sugar intake by at least half and salt consumption by 50 to 80%.

They recommend that by "hiding the salt shaker and the sugar bowl," seniors can cut down and still enjoy their foods by using spices and herbs as substitutes.

There is much that seniors, both men and women, can do to help themselves with food buying and meal planning. Labels are a big plus, but they can't help you if you don't read them. Do you know the different grades of canned goods? There are standard, fancy and choice grades, and each one is higher than the other in price. Remember, too, that bigger isn't necessarily cheaper if storage is a problem. Wasting a product through spoilage helps no one, not even the garbageman—he just has more work to do.

Men, especially those living alone, have more problems than women in the cooking field, so the Senior Citizens in Ithaca, N.Y. decided to do something about it. They not only held cooking classes for men, they also put out a cookbook with a positive approach to eating alone and liking it. To go along with cooking procedures, they put little ditties beside each recipe:

Carrots are yellow and spinach is green.

They both help produce the skin of a queen.

Education in nutrition is there for the asking; all levels of government have pamphlets on eating habits and how to improve them. Library shelves are filled with how-to books, and if a senior is stumped, he or she can always ask the family or a neighbor.

Because they lack practice in the kitchen, many men are like Joe, who sheepishly confessed, "When my wife went to the hospital, I couldn't even make a good cup of coffee." Now armed with a good basic cookbook and some telephone coaching from his daughter, he can "turn out a half-decent meal."

Joe's friend across the hall in his high-rise is also a "chief cook and bottle washer." He relies heavily, though, on packaged foods. This man finds that although they are more costly, they offer variety and are certainly superior to his own cooking.

Both men have trouble coping with all the propaganda about foods—what is fact and what is fiction? Food fads form the basis of a major industry and older people are as gullible as their grandchildren.

Being overweight (too many seniors have this problem) makes us vulnerable to crash diets, especially liquid protein. Many articles advertise the success stories, few tell the tales of disaster.

This problem has become so acute that the Canadian government has taken action to warn consumers against using these products as their only source of food. The Food and Drug Act, as amended Section B.01.033, January 1978, states that all such foods sold in Canada must carry on the label: "Caution—Do not use as sole source of nutrition."

The United States, however, relies on the protection of the First Amendment. "If the label on a food product makes false or misleading claims, the Food and Drug Administration of the U.S. Department of Health, Education and Welfare, can take action on the grounds that the product is mislabeled or misbranded."

Promotions for fad foods or diets often do not make any direct claims; they refer to a book, pamphlet, speech or magazine, and thus, these indirect promotions receive the protection of the First Amendment to the Constitution of the United States.

Scientific rebuttal of food and nutrition myths published and perpetuated in faddist literature is futile, because almost daily we are besieged by new claims of "no aging" diets and "eat more and weigh less" plans. There is no magic in any specific food item; our bodies need a proper balance of all nutrients.

Over the past few years Vitamin E sales have soared. Why? Because it has been claimed Vitamin E will grow hair, ease arthritis, prevent ulcers and make

a senior sexually young. Dr. Edward H. Rynearson, recently retired from the Mayo Clinic, has said, "Americans love hogwash." and that is just what these claims
are—hogwash!

Sometimes, it is not so much what we eat as what
we don't eat. Often with our older population it is the
stimulus which creates appetite that is lacking. People
who live alone hate to eat alone and so resort to the
"tea and toast" syndrome. They need an incentive to
eat well.

This lack of appetite can sometimes be helped by
dressing up one's surroundings, by listening to good
music, by making mealtime a special part of the day.
Eating out, even at Woolworth's, can be a real treat.

In a few communities, school cafeterias have been
opened to seniors; after the student rush is over, the
staff looks after the older citizens. True, it makes for
longer days for those in the kitchen, but most don't
mind when they are compensated in their pay checks,
and the nutritional health of seniors is vastly improved, thus cutting medical costs.

There are also volunteer projects like Meals-on-
Wheels. Over 400 are now in operation in the United
States, with their equivalent in Canada delivering hot
meals to elderly people who have difficulty in preparing their own food.

Some high-rise senior complexes have their own
cafeteria; others have pot-luck meals once a week in
the lounge area. If these programs don't exist where
you live, invite someone in and start your own plan. It
is surprising how appetites perk up when there's company. By changing their nutritional lifestyle, those on
the senior side can add quality to their years by—eating well, feeling well and being well.

THE BENEFITS GOOD NUTRITION BRINGS

Good eating habits make a difference to your health and vitality and, it's never too late to reap the benefits that balanced nutrition can bring. Whether you are six or sixty your body requires the essential nutrients that a variety of food provides.

To keep healthy and to look and feel your best, choose many different foods from each of the Four Food Groups everyday.

CANADA'S FOOD GUIDE FOR SENIORS

FOOD GROUPS	DAILY NEEDS	HINTS FOR THE CALORIE CONSCIOUS
MILK AND MILK PRODUCTS 2 SERVINGS Skim, 2%, whole, buttermilk, reconstituted dry or evaporated milk, yogurt, cheese, cottage cheese are included in the Milk Group.	Examples of one serving: 1 cup (250 mL) milk, yogurt, or cottage cheese 1½ oz (45g) cheese	Plain yogurt has less sugar than the fruit flavored variety. Try buying plain yogurt and adding unsweetened or fresh fruit to it. - Try some of the skim milk cheeses that are available or other low fat cheeses, such as Mozarella and Edam.
MEAT AND ALTERNATES 2 SERVINGS Meat, fish, poultry, beans, peas, lentils, nuts, seeds, cheese and eggs are included in the Meat and Alternates Group.	Examples of one serving: 2-3 oz. (60-90g) cooked lean meat, poultry, liver, or fish 4 tbsp. (60 mL) peanut butter 1 cup (250 mL) cooked dried peas, beans or lentils ⅓-1 cup (80-250 mL) nuts or seeds 2 oz. (60g) cheese 2 eggs,	- Use cooking methods that help to remove fat, such as baking, broiling or boiling. - Choose lean cuts of meat and trim off visible fat. - Poultry and fish contain less fat than other meats. Remember to remove the skin from poultry before eating. That's where most of the fat is found. - Drain oil from canned fish before eating.

FRUITS AND VEGETABLES

4-5 SERVINGS

Include at least 2 vegetables. All fruits and vegetables, cooked raw and their juices are included in the Fruit and Vegetable Group.

Examples of one serving:

1/2 cup (125 mL) vegetables or fruit
1/2 cup (125 mL) juice
1 medium raw vegetable or fresh fruit

- Eat vegetables with spices and lemon juice, rather than with butter and sauces.

- Use unsweetened rather than sweetened juices.

- Buy water packed fruit or fruit canned in its own juice.

- Look for frozen unsweetened fruits.

- Serve potatoes baked or boiled, rather than fried.

BREAD AND CEREALS

3-5 SERVINGS

Any whole-grain or enriched bread, cereal, or pasta (rice, macaroni, noodles, spaghetti) are included in the Bread and Cereal Group.

Examples of one serving:

1 slice bread
1/2-1 cup cooked or ready-to-eat cereal
1 roll or muffin
1/2-3/4 cup pasta (noodles, rice, spaghetti)

- Be careful about how much you add to breads and cereals in terms of spreads, or sweeteners, such as honey, jams or jellies.

- Unsweetened whole grain cereals and breads rather than sweet rolls or doughnuts are your best choices.

A GUIDE FOR EVERY DAY

FRUIT

2 servings of fruit or juice including a satisfactory source of Vitamin C e.g. oranges, tomatoes, vitaminized apple juice.

VEGETABLES

1 serving of potatoes
2 servings of other vegetables preferably yellow or green and often raw.

MILK and MILK PRODUCTS

1½ cups of milk etc.

1 cup milk· = 1 oz. cheddar cheese
           2 oz. processed cheese
           3 scoops of ice cream
           1 cup cottage cheese, or
           1 cup yogurt

MEAT and FISH

1 serving of meat, fish or poultry
eat liver occasionally
eggs, cheese, dried beans or peas may be used in place of meat
In addition eggs and cheese each at least 3 times a week.

CEREAL and BREAD

1 serving of whole grain cereal
bread (with butter or fortified margarine)

Protection
Repair   are
Energy

3 good reasons
to eat well every
day.

Check yourself

Fruit
2 servings

Vegetables
1 serving potato
2 servings other

Milk etc.
1½ cups

Meats etc.
1 serving

Cereal
1 serving
cereal bread

HOW DOES THIS MENU MATCH UP TO CANADA'S FOOD GUIDE FOR SENIORS?

2 Meats and Alternates
  — meat loaf
  — cheese

2 Milk and Milk Products
  — milk pudding
  — milk on cereal
  — cocoa made with milk

3-5 Breads and Cereals
  — hot or cold cereal
  — muffin
  — toast

4-5 Fruits and Vegetables
  — apple juice
  — potato
  — banana
  — vegetable soup
  — mushrooms
  — broccoli
  — pear

A perfect score!

If you are more active in the afternoon than in the evening, why not have your main meal of the day at noon, and a lighter evening meal?

Whatever meal pattern works best for *you* is the right one—just as long as you meet the recommendations set out in Canada's Food Guide by the end of the day.

A day's meal plan could look something like this:

Sample Menu For a Day

BREAKFAST

Hot or cold cereal with milk, apple juice, coffee or tea

MORNING SNACK
(Eat this with breakfast instead, if desired)

Bran muffin with cheese

DINNER
(At noon, the best time for a complete meal)

Individual meat-loaf
Small baked potato
Broccoli
Milk pudding

AFTERNOON SNACK
(Or instead of an afternoon snack, have this with supper)

Pear

A LIGHT SUPPER
(Preferred by many)

Vegetable soup
Creamed peas on toast sprinkled with grated cheese

BEDTIME SNACK
(To fill in gaps check Canada's Food Guide)

Banana
Cocoa made with milk

A few extra reminders:

Try to plan menus for one week at a time.
Choose the main protein dish first, from the meats and alternates group (e.g. baked beans). Then choose accompaniments from the other three food groups.

Fruits and Vegetables (e.g. tossed salad and banana for dessert)
Milk and Milk Products (e.g. glass of milk)
Breads and Cereals (e.g. toast)

Exercise

Gerontologists tell us that exercise is the closest thing we have to the fountain of youth. They claim we don't wear out, we rust out!

It's obvious everyone can't be an athlete, but that doesn't mean we can't be physically fit. The greatest saboteur of good health is inactivity, both mental and physical. When muscles aren't used, they lose their strength and elasticity; they become soft and flabby.

Exercise for health is not a new concept. In fact, Charles Dickens said, "The sum of the whole is this: walk and be happy; walk and be healthy." This 19th century novelist believed that walking steadily and with a purpose is "the best way to lengthen our days."

Walking is our biggest fitness bargain. It is the cheapest exercise in terms of time, money and energy. All you really need is a good pair of shoes.

Walking can be a joy; anyone who makes it their regular form of exercise will be amazed at the pleasure and satisfaction it can bring. However, the first few times out are definitely going to be an effort—like work, it isn't easy at first. There are going to be a few sore muscles too; after all, some of them have been in hibernation for a long time.

Martin was a retired drill press operator. One afternoon, his spirits sagging, bored, he decided he had to do something! He took up walking. The first day, he walked four miles one way. When he got to the other side of town he was beat, and he had to take a taxi home. The next day he stayed in bed all day; he ached all over.

Seniors who are going to make walking a part of their daily routine must remember to walk only a modest distance that first day, and then only a little farther the second, because there is always the coming-back.

Walking shouldn't overtax you, but just ambling or sauntering won't do! A senior must walk at a reasonably brisk pace to get the full benefit from a walking program. The average pace should be about 3½ miles per hour, but the time spent walking at that speed should be built up gradually from 10 minutes to 45 minutes or so.

Walking can ease tension, frustration and nervousness. Leonard, for example, was a chemist before he retired, and he found his new lifestyle hard to take. When he started walking, he said, "My frustrations and tensions seemed to flow out of my fingertips." Do you have trouble getting a good night's sleep? Leonard does most of his walking in the late afternoon or evening and he says, "Now, at bedtime I don't need an aspirin or tranquilizer; I'm tired and I can sleep."

Most seniors don't like to go out in bad weather, but one walking enthusiast says she likes the soft splashes of spring rain, the velvet touch of snow and the wild challenge of cold and wind against her cheek. "Human beings have been walking for a million years and maybe more, depending when life began," she says, "and the weather never stopped them—why should it stop us?"

Even with all the physical benefits and pleasures of walking, there are a few dangers too—every safety precaution must be taken. Seniors need to remember that although they may be physically fit, they are not quite as quick on their feet as they used to be, so it is sound advice to cross streets only at intersections or designated crosswalks. Even then, look before you cross—and then look again!

For those using country roads or lanes, always walk facing the traffic. Don't let cars sneak up from behind, and wear bright colored clothing so they can see you. Walk defensively; if you're in a contest with a car, you certainly won't come out the winner.

Walking can put zest back into a tired old life, but knowing and doing are two different things. For those who for physical or personal reasons do not like walking, there are many other forms of exercise just as beneficial. Some of these leisure sports date back as far as the early Egyptians.

Lawn bowling is one of them, and it doesn't matter if you're a single, pair or trio, widow or widower, odd numbers aren't out of place.

Sir Francis Drake was so absorbed by lawn bowling that when he was told the Spanish Armada had been sighted, he said, "I'll finish this game first, then I'll defeat the Spaniards."

In the 16th century, lawn bowling was considered the national sport of Scotland and was brought across the ocean by the early settlers.

The average lawn bowler walks about a mile per game, lifting and rolling a 3½-pound bowl (not a ball) approximately 42 times. There are some other advantages besides the fresh air and mental stimulation.

"You can't leave your brains at home if you want to play a good game," said one senior who was in competition for a gold cup.

The mechanics of the game are quite simple: there are one to four members on a team, and the two opposing teams bowl alternately to see how close they can come to the jack, a white earthen bowl rolled down the green at the start of the game. One point is scored by each team member who puts his or her bowl closer to the jack than that of the opposing team. Games usually consist of 12 to 21 ends or plays.

Do you feel you're too old to play? George Balkwill started to lawn bowl when he was 70. At 93, he took the high score at his local lawn bowling green.

Besides being stimulating, the sport offers the challenge of competition and the thrill of winning. And there's an added benefit—plenty of good companionship.

Swimming is another exercise many seniors enjoy. The therapeutic value of moving in water is unquestionably high, because it soothes and loosens up stiff old joints. What about those who can't swim and those who are afraid of the water? Well, it's never too late. Just get a bathing suit and enrol in the nearest class.

"One thing about being in a senior's swim class, we all bulge in the wrong places, so we don't have to be embarrassed by our sagging waistlines," a former non-swimmer said.

Rita Lutz, a swimming instructor and a senior citizen, says that one of the main problems in teaching older persons to swim is to get them to trust the water. Rita starts all non-swimmers on a back float. This provides a restful position in the water and allows for easier breathing—many seniors have breathing problems. Rita also insists on good body posture which she believes makes swimming easier.

"One man who has really had to persevere was caught under a water wheel in England when he was a boy. He's really up-tight, but he's staying with the program, and what's more, he will receive his certificate with the rest of the class."

The ages in Rita Lutz's swimming classes vary from 58 to 83 and over 65% were non-swimmers before they started.

Bicycling is another way seniors can keep fit. Although in many areas cyclists can only enjoy eight months or so of rideable weather, bicycling still has much to offer. It's a cheap means of transportation, bicycles are noise- and pollution-free, and the exercise it takes to pedal them improves health.

One 78 year old says, "I cycle three miles every morning before breakfast. It peps up my appetite and puts me into a good frame of mind for the rest of the day."

There are also some financial benefits to riding a bicycle. The cost of a mechanic's labor to repair a car is approximately $18 an hour. Often bicycle owners with a little know-how can do the job themselves.

Many seniors who feel a bit shaky on a two-wheeler have gone to the adult tricycle which costs about $250. Although busy city streets are not conducive to bicycle riding, people in suburbs, villages and small communities have it made.

Bicycling is a stimulating exercise, but like all active exercises, moderation is the key. It is not sensible to buy a bike one day and pedal for six miles the next; a gradual build-up from a half mile to a greater distance is better for you.

Like swimming and walking, bicycling relieves tension, reduces joint stiffness, reduces the fat in the body tissue and lessens the fatigue level. In addition, various organs and systems of the body, particularly the digestive system, are stimulated through activity and as a result, work more effectively.

For those who like to cycle in the privacy of their own homes, there are exercise bikes, but unfortunately, fresh air is not included.

A bicycle is not a toy; it is a lawful vehicle subject to the laws of the road, and like other vehicles, comes under the authority of highway traffic acts. Cyclists must stop at stop signs, go the proper way on a one-way street, signal when making a turn and wait for a green light. Reflectors are mandatory for all units, and anyone riding at night must have a light.

According to one policeman, "You can get a ticket for speeding." But he says they're rare, especially for those on the senior side. A 10-speed bicycle, though, is capable of doing 35 miles an hour in a 25 m.p.h. zone.

Are senior bicyclists more accident-prone than their younger counterparts? From the meagre statistics available, the answer is no; in fact, many communities have never had a bicycle accident involving a senior citizen.

In these days of high inflation and skyrocketing energy costs, bicycling is a practical way to build up our fitness bank accounts as well as our financial ones.

Another way to build up your fitness account is by skating. Jack Lawson started skating when he was five; he swung into figure skating at 35 and began stilt-skating a few years later. Now on the threshold of his 80th birthday, he looks more like a man of 60, and is more supple than most men of 40.

Not content to just skate, this man each year builds his own 60-by-100-foot outdoor rink. He also makes boot adjustments for young skaters as well as taking part, along with his young partner Mary Penny, in numerous ice skating follies and reviews. Jack believes in the theory of mind over matter, and once when he broke his leg, he fashioned a skate for his cast, and despite doctor's orders, went skating. Later, the doctor admitted it was the best thing he could have done, because now Jack has no stiffness or arthritis.

For 57 years he was a barber, and has now transferred this full-time job to a part-time one in the foyer of his own home. In the summer, in place of skating, he gardens. Refusing to use mechanical tools, he sticks to the traditional hoe and rake.

All across the land seniors are gardening, for fun, for exercise and to ease the pinch of the sinking value of the dollar. People in high-rise apartments are renting land for gardening, and sometimes they are lucky enough to get it free in return for keeping the land clean. It is the exercise value that takes gardening beyond dollars and cents. It can rejuvenate old muscles, but it can also bring on a heart attack. Moderation, knowing one's limitations, is the key.

Now, even in nursing homes and homes for the aged, exercise programs are being introduced. Fitness programs for people over 60 are being promoted by activity directors and therapists from coast to coast. They are proving that exercise gives a much-needed sense of well-being and fitness to the senior citizen, regardless of his or her place of residence.

There are no miracle drugs to keep us young, but exercise is the closest thing we have to making old bodies young again.

Physical Losses

There are five physical losses a senior can suffer before or after age 65. They relate to eyes, ears, teeth, feet and joints, all crucial to our defense system against the impairments of aging and which need to be guarded well. When we have problems in one or more of these areas, the whole quality of our lives is affected.

They are basic to our mobility and to our health, yet we slight them, ignore them, subject them to all sorts of ridiculous "cures." Not until we lose them do we realize their value.

Eyes: Statistics show that 50% of the blind in Canada are over 60 years of age; the Canadian National Institute for the Blind states that half such cases could be prevented. Our eyes are one of our main lines of defense, so why do so many seniors fail to treat them with respect?

Older people sometimes do not go to a doctor when they have blurred vision, spots before their eyes and other usual aches and pains. They have been brainwashed to believe these are symptoms of growing old. Our eyes age, just as our bodies do, and some deterioration of our vision may occur, but early detection is still the key to preventing and curing cataracts, glaucoma and macular degeneration, the latter now being the most prevalent.

The macula is the most sensitive spot in the retina. It is used for seeing the fine detail when reading, writing and watching TV. When this central function becomes impaired, the condition is called macular degeneration. With the help of "low visual aids" many people who are experiencing this hardening of the arteries behind the retina can continue all their usual activities. Actually, when the macula, the fine tuner of the eye, is affected, the peripheral field (outer border area) usually escapes the vision problem.

After an eye examination, when someone says, "I have presbyopia!" all kinds of dark ills are conjured up. Presbyopia is common to people over 40. "When you see someone reading the newspaper at arm's length, then you know he or she has presbyopia," an eye specialist said at a seminar on problems of aging.

Glasses prescribed by an optometrist can correct the problem. Presbyopia is simply the inability of the eye to focus on objects close by; usually the same person can see things a mile away.

Some seniors limit their eye use because they erroneously believe they will injure their eyes by overworking them. R. W. Kennedy, the administrator of the London Branch of the Canadian National Institute for the Blind, said, "We can't hurt our eyes by using them. Reading or sewing too much or watching TV can fatigue the eyes, but it will never hurt their vision."

Diabetic retinaopathy is now emerging as one of the main causes of blindness. Diabetes is a disease which affects all the tissue of the body, including the fine blood vessels inside the eye, making them more fragile and more likely to bleed. Eye care is an integral part of the care of diabetes, and each diabetic should be under close, regular medical supervision.

A cataract, another cause of blindness, occurs when the normal lens of the eye becomes cloudy. The most common are "senile cataracts," found in people past middle age, and since they are somewhat related to age, as our life span increases, so does the problem.

Many doctors of the old school have their patients wait "for the cataracts to ripen." Many young specialists hold to the theory that early detection and early surgery, done under a general or local anesthesia, give the best results.

Surgery, though, leaves a patient without a lens so either a plastic lens or glasses must be used to give sight back to the impaired eye.

When a patient is released from hospital after surgery, drops must be put into the eyes each day, and under no circumstances is the patient to bend or bang his or her head. For seniors living alone, this can present quite a problem. Many homes for the aged will not accept patients for a week or ten days to help them over this delicate care period. But the Victorian Order of Nurses and other public health nurses will make visiting a cataract patient a part of their schedule.

Wiggling spots before the eyes are not usually cause for alarm, but if those spots appear in showers, along with flashes of light and decreased vision, that's an entirely different story. When this happens, people assume they have glaucoma, and are petrified with fear, instead of having the symptoms checked and their fears allayed.

Chronic glaucoma is a disturbance in the optic nerve, and is associated with increased pressure inside the eyeball. It is not cancerous or infectious, and if diagnosed early, can be arrested without further loss of vision. It is important to identify glaucoma early, and this can only be done by regular check-ups.

Ears: A hearing loss is not necessarily a sign of old age, but the aging process is directly related to loss of hearing, although there are many reasons for this loss: ear infection, head injuries, tumors, exposure to loud noises and reactions to drugs.

The National Council of Senior Citizens was recently told by Attorney David H. Marlin, National Director of Legal Research and Services for the Elderly that more than 14.5 million Americans have some type of hearing problem. One in 40 has an impairment serious enough to affect communications with others, and these hearing problems affect four out of every 10 persons 75 years of age and over.

Loss of hearing is an insidious disease, creeping up on its victims, an invisible handicap. Before they realize it, communication has become a serious problem—not just communication with others, the whole world of sound has been turned off. Sometimes, because someone has caught a few words or a phrase, meaning is taken out of context, wrong things are said, and friendships are lost. When this happens, people retreat into themselves and more barriers go up. For many seniors living alone, TV is a magic world of communication which brings pleasure and information. It too is removed from a senior's reach by lack of sound.

How do you know if you have a hearing problem? There are six fairly common patterns:

1). Do you frequently ask companions to repeat what they have said?

2). Do you have difficulty understanding conversation in a noisy place?

3). Do you find your attention wandering when people are talking to you?

4). Do you often ask that the radio or TV be turned up and then discover from faces of other listeners that it is too loud?

5). Do you have frequent ear infections, dizziness, constant ringing in the ears?

6). Do you have to listen closely to hear what is going on, and find that this extreme concentration is fatiguing?

Like so many of our problems, we try to ignore loss of hearing. When we can't ignore it, we conceal it. We have to face loss of hearing squarely, then do something about it.

Otologists (ear specialists) and otolaryngologists (ear, nose and throat specialists) can give advice and aid. Unfortunately, there are a few who take advantage of a senior's hearing problem, and sell them new, revolutionary hearing aids that will help them regain their hearing. In spite of what a salesperson says, there is no such device. Many of these so-called salespeople work on commission, and seniors are gullible customers because of their fear of deafness. A hearing aid costs anywhere from $200 to $700, and binaural systems cost almost twice as much.

Hearing aids are no longer cumbersome boxes strapped to the chest, but minute transistors that pick up all sounds, both desirable and undesirable. It is often wise to rent a hearing aid before buying. This rental fee, in most cases, can later be applied to the full purchase price of the aid, should you decide to buy.

The Better Business Bureau has come up with a list of what a senior should accept in a hearing aid. First, the quality of sound should be good. This will help the recipient hear speech in both quiet and noisy places. Some seniors purchase aids and never wear them because they are not comfortable or cause confusion when amplifying and controlling sound. Second, it should be comfortable. Then, besides the initial cost of purchase, other costs must be considered: is the ear mold included with the set? How costly is the upkeep? Is the set durable, or will another purchase be necessary in a few years?

Not all your hearing problems can be helped by a hearing aid. Your ear specialist or family doctor will have that information for you. Armed with that knowledge, you can proceed to buy or to not buy.

Teeth: Good teeth and dentures also play a big part in a senior's well-being and health. The problem, though, is not always the teeth and dentures, but also the gums and supporting tissues.

Tooth decay is not due to aging. Our teeth are made to last a lifetime; poor dietary habits, neglect of dental hygiene, infection and injury are the culprits.

Most seniors, though, lose their teeth through periodontal diseases, more commonly called pyorrhea. Pyorrhea is marked by the progressive destruction of the supporting gum tissue, accompanied by formation of pus; without treatment this can become so painful that all the teeth have to be removed. For seniors who elect to go without dentures afterwards, additional harm can be caused to the muscles and ligaments involved in chewing.

Years ago it was standard procedure, if older people were having problems with their teeth, to remove them. Today, extraction is only used when all else fails. Dr. David Banting of the Department of Social Dentistry, University of Western Ontario at London, stresses, "Too often, getting all a senior's teeth pulled isn't the end of the problem, it's just the beginning."

Now dentists will try to save at least one tooth, or even just a root. "This gives us something to clamp the denture onto, especially on the lower jaw," Banting added.

Many older people's mouth problems are caused by ill-fitting dentures. Not everyone, though, has been as embarrassed as the senior who sneezed at a banquet: "My teeth just flew right out! And where did they land? Right in the jellied salad!" Chewing is the first step in our digestive process, and when our mouths are tender from gum sores, often caused by ill-fitting dentures, we tend to eat softer foods that contain more starch. Apples, celery, carrot sticks and pears, all rich in nutrients we need, must be passed by.

Unfortunately, seniors don't visit their dentists regularly enough, especially those who have dentures, but dentures, like their users, grow old too, and need to be refitted. Also, in later life the shape of the mouth may change rapidly, and if the change is drastic enough, new dentures may be the only answer.

Another problem that tends to become more frequent with age is cavities on the roots of teeth. They don't develop overnight, though; they're helped along by years of neglect and improper care. Gums shrink, exposing the teeth, and cavities begin. By the time we reach 40, if our teeth have not been properly cared for, root exposure is under way. By the time we reach 60, root exposure is on a runaway course.

Myths seem to build up about the teeth, and contrary to public opinion, less than 1 per cent of senior's mouth problems are cancerous.

In many rural communities, dentists are scarce and there is little financial help available for seniors for dental care, so many go without. Consequently, when they must go to a clinic, their minor problems have grown into major ones. There are many simple things older persons can do to help themselves, like removing dentures at night. "This allows the tissue underneath the dentures to recuperate or rest," says Dr. Banting. "And this is a good time to thoroughly clean, not just rinse, the mouth and dentures." He went on to say that fittings should be kept in water overnight, as they have a tendency to dry out and change shape.

Feet: If teeth are the first step toward a good digestion, then our feet are the main defensive line against curtailed mobility. Yet people really don't appreciate their feet until they become older and have difficulty getting around; looking after one's feet, though, isn't always as simple as it sounds. Because of arthritis and other aging problems that make joints stiff and bending impossible, some seniors haven't seen their feet in years.

As we grow older our toenails have a tendency to thicken. If a senior can't do it for himself, a podiatrist or health nurse can buff these down, keeping them thin so they don't develop an out-of-proportion thickness.

Sores between the toes are also not an uncommon foot problem for seniors. Skin becomes dry and tends to crack, and where a break occurs, germs love to congregate. A lubricant like lanolin can satisfactorily solve the problem. Sometimes, too, when we bathe, we forget our feet and don't wash and dry them carefully enough, especially between the toes.

One 79-year-old woman told her podiatrist, "When I walk, my feet feel like they are on fire." To remedy the situation, all that was really needed was a heavier sock; quite an easy solution for men, but not so easy for women who are a little more style-conscious. One woman solved her problem by wearing a cotton sockette inside her nylons. The sockette was low enough that it didn't show above her shoes, and absorbent enough to take the perspiration that was causing the burning in her feet.

Dr. Emily Newell of the podiatric clinic at St. Joseph's Hospital says, "Most foot problems are

Lynda Middleton

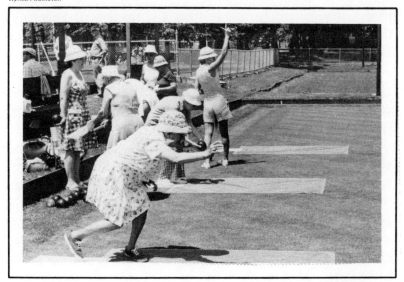

caused by shoes. Too often we try to get our feet to fit the shoes, when it should be the shoes that fit the feet." According to Dr. Newell, almost 80% of all foot problems are caused by shoes.

The basic reason we wear shoes is to protect our feet, so if your feet are problem-free, a senior can choose any type of shoe that is comfortable. "Our feet change with age," says Dr. Newell. "They get wider; if you used to take a size five, don't be surprised if at age 70 you are taking a size or two larger.

The correct shoe size is important. Tight-fitting shoes can cause bunions, corns and other related problems. Therefore, when a senior's feet are measured for size, he or she should be standing on them. The widest part of the foot is the ball where the big toe begins. From the heel to the ball of the foot is two-thirds of the length of our foot; from the ball to the tip of our toes is another third.

Dr. Newell stresses that seniors should not let a salesman talk them into taking a longer length of shoe just to get the width. Some people have longer arches

79

than others, and by accepting a shoe that is too long, their feet can be thrown out of proper balance. Shoe size doesn't really make any difference, except to the ego; it is the measurement of the foot that is important, and numbers are only a handy guide—there is a great difference among Canadian, American and European systems of sizing.

When buying shoes it is important to remember that leather will stretch; vinyl and plastic will not retain its stretch. If a senior has a corn or bad stress area, a leather shoe can be stretched over that particular spot, and extra room achieved. If a salesman stretches a plastic or vinyl shoe, once off the foot, it will revert to its old shape, and the stress area will still be a possible source of pain.

Often seniors who have flat feet are told to get arch supports. Podiatrists advise that as long as the condition is painless, forget it. However, if a senior is experiencing pain, then, *upon professional advice*, he or she might be told to get arch supports. These supports vary drastically in price and material: little foam inserts from a drug store are less than a dollar, while steel ones range in price from $38 to $150.

Your feet are precious, so if you're having major problems, consult a doctor; don't be "a fool" and prescribe for yourself.

Creaking bones and stiffening joints: These have long been associated with old age; although collectively a major health problem, they do not rank high as a cause of death. They are high, however, on the quackery list, especially arthritis, inflammation of a joint.

Arthritis is not one disease but a variety of rheumatic diseases, the most common being rheumatoid arthritis, osteoarthritis and gout. Our best defense against these chronic diseases is early diagnosis and treatment.

Rheumatoid arthritis is a systemic disease which affects not only the joints but the body as well, and the usual treatment prescribed by doctors is rest, therapeutic exercise and medication.

Osteoarthritis, more commonly called degenerative joint disease, affects 97% of those 60 years of age and over. It is the wearing-out of the cartilage covering the weight-bearing joints.

"Treatment beneficial to one kind of arthritis may be useless or even harmful for another," says a member of the Arthritis Society. And because of their very natures—symptoms wax and wane with intermittent periods of remission—the diseases lend themselves to quack cures. Last year in Canada alone seniors spent over $100 million on fraudulent cures.

While heat has been used for over 2000 years to comfort arthritic pain, last year when a South African heart surgeon used and recommended a special heating pad, hundreds of consumers lined up to buy them at $70 each. Yet these pads had no special properties for arthritic sufferers.

It is natural for people to want relief from their pain, but wearing copper bracelets or gold coins, using vibrators or other electronic devices are not going to cure arthritis. Some seniors are turning to health foods such as alfalfa tablets, although medical research has proven that foods do not play a role in causing these diseases.

While most of these bogus remedies are harmless, the Arthritis Society warns that the danger lies in the long run, if the quack cure prevents the sufferer from receiving proper treatment before irreversible damage to the joints is done.

It is ironic that for every dollar spent on research, $25 will be spent on miracle cures, yet research holds the only answer.

Senility, Alcoholism and Drug Abuse

One of the greatest fears of our elderly is senility. It is a term used excessively by professionals and lay people alike to explain the behavior and condition of a person 65 or over, whose mind wanders, whose thoughts aren't coherent and who appears to be retreating from reality. These symptoms, erroneously called "senility" are glibly blamed on a single cause: aging.

Dr. Ronald Cape, coordinator of geriatric medicine at the University of Western Ontario at London, Ontario, states, "There is no such thing as senility. There is, however, a disease called senile dementia which can sometimes affect the elderly."

Senile dementia is a malfunction in the brain, a degenerative change in brain cells. From biochemical studies geriatricians are hoping to replace with drugs the loss of substances that prevent these malfunctions. But progress in this area is slow, and success is still about five years down the road.

Because "senility" has become such a catch-all for loss of memory, irritability and confusion, people fail to look for the real causes of these symptoms. Unfortunately, society itself produces the chief causes: depression, loneliness and inactivity of the mind and the body. When seniors feel life is not worth living, it becomes so, and they withdraw into themselves.

Less than 13% of patients admitted to hospitals for mental disorders suffer from senility. But 49% do suffer from depression caused by a feeling of worthlessness, dissatisfaction and unhappiness. "Most of the problems of the aged, such as 'senility' are caused by poor environment rather than organic breakdown," says Vera McIver of the Juan de Fuca Hospital Society.

In most cases, this wrongly labeled condition is reversible through proper medication, diet, psychotherapy and a better environment. It is not the dragon it once was.

Alcoholism, though, is fast taking its place as a problem of the elderly. And it's not just the poor who are stumbling—middle class and the higher income people are also falling prey to this "disease." Alcoholism *is* a disease, a disease of loneliness and boredom.

Few problems will drag a senior down quicker than alcoholism. This is due partly to physical tolerance—a senior's physical tolerance for alcohol decreases as his or her stresses of living increase. These stresses take many forms; for people like Mae, it was being on her own for the first time in her life. She and her husband Frank had gone everywhere together for 34 years. Suddenly she was alone and afraid, so to buck up her courage she took a drink, and soon the one became two and the two became three. Before long she was drinking instead of eating.

One morning she awoke to find herself on the floor; her collarbone was broken. Later, her doctor encouraged her to seek help for her problem, but she was reluctant—an alcoholic at her age? Never! "Besides, I only use it to relax," she said. Alcohol, though, has other properties. It is an analgesic and depressant, and seniors are particularly susceptible to these effects.

"The fact that alcohol is a drug comes as a surprise to many people," said a member of Alcoholics Anonymous who works with seniors. "Maybe that is due to the fact it has been with us for such a long time." (The first known brewery was in operation in Egypt in 3700 BC.)

Joe was a typical candidate for alcoholism. He was troubled with arthritis and had difficulty getting about, he lived on a farm, had a better-than-average income and after his wife died he found the time heavy on his hands. So he drank to relieve the restrictedness of his activities and the endless boredom.

When his daughter came for a visit she noticed his excessive drinking. She took the matter to her brother who lived close by, but he only shrugged and said, "So the old boy drinks too much—what's the harm? It's one of the few pleasures he has left."

Many families choose to do nothing when they find that a parent has turned to the bottle. Others are completely unaware of the fact their mother or father is having difficulties with alcohol.

Alcoholics, especially senior alcoholics, are a relatively hidden group. They usually live alone, they are rarely arrested for driving when intoxicated, and since they are usually retired, they don't have problems at work. When friends notice they have a slight memory lapse or are a little unsteady on their feet, they simply relate it to the aging process. The physical symptoms of alcoholism can be easily confused with the symptoms of "senility."

The alcohol problem is not only confined to seniors living alone in isolated areas, it is extremely prevalent in retirement settlements. Social activities in these communities, designed especially for seniors, are conducive to heavy drinking. "We play bridge, we have a drink; we play golf, we have a drink; we sit and chat, we have a drink," said a retired engineer, who found himself an alcoholic after three years of the "good life."

Another man, a 78 year old and a recovered alcoholic, expressed his feelings about his life at the retirement settlement this way: "There is just so much golfing, fishing and traveling a person can do before he goes off the deep end." This man now spends his time as a volunteer helping others to lick the same problem he experienced.

The senior drinker usually falls into one of two categories. First, there are those who drank excessively before retirement and now, to fill their increased leisure, have increased their drinking. And then there are the others who drank only a little before retirement or bereavement, but have now turned to alcohol and are using it as a crutch to face social and psychological problems.

Many seniors feel that "a meal without wine is like a day without sunshine," and most scientists feel a sensible use of alcohol won't harm you. In fact, it can relieve tension and bring a little cheer. However, it does contain calories, and these calories slide down so easily. One drink can stimulate an appetite, but too many drinks can overtake it. Alcohol abuse and malnutrition go hand in hand.

There are few specialized services to deal with geriatric alcoholism. Doctors are often reluctant to put "alcoholism" on a patient's card—many institutions will not accept patients who have a chronic alcohol problem, because they're too hard to manage.

Sadly, the wide-ranging problems seniors experience due to excessive use of alcohol are matched by those resulting from excessive use of drugs. Too often, seniors rely on pills and medicines, while not giving serious thought as to why they are taking them.

Actually, a drug is a substance that by its chemical nature can alter the structure or function of the body, and they have been with us for a long time. Opium was used in Mesopotamia in the year 5000 BC, according to ancient records.

We use drugs indiscriminately and are becoming a drugged society. Right now there are over 700 basic chemical compounds on the prescription market, and these have well over 20,000 brand names.

Drugs are a godsend when properly used. They can combat infection and pain, restore a healthy chemical balance or bolster faltering body processes. But when they are misused or used ignorantly, they become a menace.

Unfortunately, many people on the senior side mishandle their medication. Some don't follow the directions typed on the bottle. Others borrow drugs from relatives and friends, with the attitude, "it helped them, so why shouldn't it help me?" Each person is different, and what is good for one senior is not good for another. There is much wisdom in the old saying, "a person who is his own doctor has a fool for a patient."

Marta was one of those fools. She had a condition, and she was given a prescription by her doctor. Although the plastic pill container had the directions pasted on it (the label showed the date and type of medication, and exactly when it should be taken), she didn't bother to read. She took the pills when she felt like it—early in the morning and late at night—even though the instructions were explicit: "take one before each meal."

For two days Marta believed she was faithfully

following her doctor's orders; yet her condition remained unchanged. So one afternoon she saw some of her husband's white pills that he had used a year ago; she decided to "doctor" herself, and she took them periodically the rest of the day.

That night her husband said, "Marta, if I didn't know you better, I'd say you were on a trip." He was right, she *was* on a trip—a trip that brought her to the hospital.

In a clinical study it was found over 66% of seniors taking drugs make mistakes in taking their prescribed medicines. This is an awesomely high percentage. What is the reason? Most often it is carelessness and thoughtlessness—just plain stupidity.

Sensitivity to drugs increases with age. When instructions say "first thing in the morning, at noon and before bed" that means the medication is to be spread out as far over the day as possible, because older people are particularly prone to feeling side effects. Often these side effects are subtle—symptoms like fatigue, insomnia or changes in type or time of bowel movement.

The National Safety Council lists barbiturates and tranquilizers as the greatest drug dangers for older people. Even the common aspirin, while fine for a cold, headache or arthritic pain, when taken in large quantities or mixed with certain other prescribed medicines, can be harmful.

An over-medicated senior can stumble or fall, break a hip (bones are brittle) or have lapses of memory. Before they know it, seniors can find themselves in a nursing home or a home for the aged.

Families and friends shouldn't be hesitant about asking questions. They should check on what a senior is taking and drinking. One of the greatest gifts we can give to those we love is a genuine concern for their health and happiness.

Safety and Crime

Keeping your life accident-free is up to you. Accidents don't just happen, they're caused. Over 53% of fatal accidents to people on the senior side occur in the home.

Why are seniors so accident prone? Failing eyesight, slower muscular coordination, loss of sense of smell, change of gait and impaired hearing are only a few of the reasons.

Since they are known problem areas, more attention should be given to these physical handicaps. Seniors must be constantly aware of their safety responsibilities if they are to lessen the number of fatal and crippling accidents.

Some accidents could be avoided: burning dinner while gossiping on the telephone; leaving objects on the stairs until the next time you go up or down; even wandering through unlit rooms. Now, with the cost of electricity on the rise, this latter type of accident is on the increase too. Seniors trip over unremembered footstools, end tables and floor ornaments—result, a broken hip.

In winter many people supplement their home heating by turning on open-flame gas heaters and stoves. Women, who often wear full-sleeved house-coats, unthinkingly reach across the flames. These sleeves easily ignite.

Some seniors like floppy slippers, or because of swollen feet, go around with their shoes untied. Joe was one of these floppy-slipper guys. Last week his right foot stepped on his left heel, and now he is nursing a twisted knee.

High on the accident source list is stairways. A handrail should be a must for any senior's home that has stairs, inside or outside—many older people have a balancing problem or an occasional moment of dizziness, and that's all it takes.

Most seniors, when they know their grand-children are coming, put everything out of harm's way. By the same logic, according to Frances McHale, supervisor of senior programs at the Forest City Kiwanis Senior Community Centre, "seniors should accident-proof their homes for their own personal safety."

Accident-proofing a house simply means seeing that stair treads have no loose, curled-up edges; rugs are non-skid; rickety chairs, no matter how comfortable, should be repaired or thrown out; no one smokes in bed; no one takes medicine in the dark—pills should be placed far enough away from the bed so that the user will have to turn on the light and be fully awake to get them.

Accidents are not inevitable. By accepting the limitations of age and making safety a personal responsibility, seniors will find that without causes, accidents just don't happen!

Personal responsibility, though, goes farther than accidents; it even enters the world of crime. There are four major types of crime affecting seniors: confidence games, consumer fraud, purse snatching and burglary.

By taking responsibility for their safety, seniors can keep from becoming victims.

Purse snatching is a crime of opportunity, so it is up to us to eliminate the opportunity. Often seniors advertise the fact they are carrying money—and senior women are more at fault than senior men. It is simply the way they handle their purses.

Mary is such a person—she advertises that she has money. How? Usually she carries her purse in her hand, hanging loosely from her fingers. After she cashes her pension check, she carries her purse in front of her stomach, or sometimes clutched close to her chest. Her overprotectiveness is blatantly advertising the fact that she is carrying more than the normal amount of cash.

Purse snatching isn't particularly a night crime; in fact, statistics show it's more frequent during the daylight hours, and is usually done by persons 19 years of age and under. Purse snatchers are very difficult to catch, mainly because of the speed at which the attack occurs. Victims, since they are approached from behind, rarely see their assailants.

How can seniors protect themselves? Certainly not by carrying a weapon, which could be turned against them. Plain common sense is their best defense; it eliminates the opportunity.

Police officers advise: "Keep to lighted areas and avoid shortcuts through parks or buildings. High shrubbery and parked vehicles also provide convenient hiding places for attackers, so beware!"

"Avoid routine!" is another piece of good advice. How many times have you heard, "I can set my watch by her"? She catches the same bus at the same corner at the same time, goes to the same bank, shops at the same stores and goes home by the same route. That woman is predictable.

Men do the same thing. And worse, often after cashing their check, they move out of line while still counting their money, and sometimes are still sorting their cash by the time they reach the street. Their wad is then stuffed into a wallet, and the wallet pushed into a hip pocket, making them prime targets for theft.

If someone grabs your purse or wallet, let them have it! Resistance can bring injury. Purse snatchers are interested in your money, not your life.

One woman who had her purse snatched reacted quite differently. She sat in the middle of the sidewalk and yelled "Fire!" Later she said, "I knew no one would come if I yelled for help, but everyone comes to a fire."

Another woman confused a would-be purse snatcher by emptying the contents of her handbag on the sidewalk as she handed it to him. This wasn't wise, but it did save her money.

Injury, often the aftermath of a snatched purse incident, can be traumatic, especially for seniors, whose bones are brittle and who are easily knocked off balance. They fall and receive concussions and broken hips, collarbones or arms. These don't easily heal. The long-term physical and psychological effects can be worse for the senior than the crime itself.

Leaving purses in shopping carts or open on a counter while you reach for something also invites theft. Actually when a woman goes shopping, all she needs is her house key, a small amount of cash (nowadays you need quite a bit—pay by check or credit card) and maybe a driver's license. If a woman does carry a purse, she should carry one with a strong clasp, one that doesn't fly open at a touch. Large basket weaves that make contents visible are also an open invitation to a thief.

What happens if you come face to face with a

burglar in your home? Play it cool. Remain motionless and don't scream. The consensus of lawmen is that "if at all possible householders should avoid confrontation with intruders."

However, there are steps you can take to protect your home and valuables. Automatic timers are an inexpensive deterrent against burglary. These devices automatically turn certain lights in your house on and off; some even turn on a radio, and light plus music gives the impression that someone is in the house.

Don't advertise your absence. Newspapers on the verandah, several quarts of milk in the box and mail sticking out of the slot are all unmistakable tips that you are away for a few days. Unmowed grass and unshoveled walks are also a giveaway. Curtains drawn for days at a time advertise no one is home.

Should you keep a gun in the house? According to police officers, "a gun in the home is far more dangerous than the threat of burglary." The National Safety Council statistics show that last year 1,200 persons were accidentally killed in their own homes and thousands more were wounded by firearms. They are not a deterrent.

A senior's best precautionary bets against purse snatching, theft and burglary are companionship, alertness and good old-fashioned common sense, plus good locks on doors and windows.

This common-sense attitude needs to be carried into the realm of the confidence man and consumer fraud. Home repairs offer a wide range of opportunity for con men. Remember when tinkers used to call at your door, sharpening knives and scissors, mending pots and pans? Other people call now, but many are not honest. They don't work for a few pennies like the tinkers, they work for hundreds of dollars, sometimes even thousands.

These fly-by-nighters usually offer a now-or-never deal, a chance of a lifetime, and they insist that the senior sign the contract immediately—no waiting until tomorrow, no thinking about it. Sign right now!

As soon as the first robin appears, it seems these con artists take to the road, offering every range of home repair from pointing-up your chimney to paving the driveway, and they don't want 5% down, they demand 50% before they begin.

This should be a tip-off in itself, but it isn't. It is not uncommon for a local tradesperson to ask for 5% of the estimated total of the bill as a binder. Quite often, when a senior is well known in the community, the tradesperson will say, "pay when the work is finished or within 30 days."

These sign-right-now deals are pressure-selling tactics, and seniors need to be suspicious. If someone can't wait for you to check with the Better Business Bureau, the Chamber of Commerce or the Consumers' Association, they are in too big a hurry, and this alone should ring a don't-get-involved bell.

If your driveway needs paving, or your foundation or roof needs repairs, call two or three local tradespeople and get estimates. If the knock-on-the-door repairer's bill is just half the local tradesperson's, there is definitely something wrong. Beware!

And if you do bite on the out-of-towner, inspect the work when it's finished; make sure it has been done properly before you make the final payment. It's better to be too careful than not careful enough.

Bankers' Associations across the continent are attempting to protect their clients with news releases telling them to beware the phony bank inspector. No matter how much this old con game is publicized, there are still a few victims who fall into the trap each year.

These fraudulent bank inspectors choose their targets carefully—usually older women who live alone. The fraud begins with a telephone call from someone posing as a bank inspector, bank examiner or bank detective. The caller claims to be investigating employee theft or tracing counterfeit bills at your bank, and because it is your bank, he would like your help. "Secrecy is the key!" He advises, "Tell no one!"

The trapper unsuspectingly becomes the trapped. As an added inducement to assisting him, the caller casually mentions that there is sure to be a reward for your cooperation. The people who get caught in this web of lies are the ones who can least afford the experience, the pensioners.

Don't take your money out of the bank for anyone! Some banks are so concerned about seniors being swindled by phony inspectors that before they release a large sum of money to you, either the manager or assistant manager will inquire about the withdrawal. They are not being nosy. They are trying to protect you, just in case.

The alone and the lonely are ripe for plucking by con artists and social swindlers. Lonely seniors need to beware of social club advertising. Dance studios that disguise their businesses as social clubs prey on the lonely. At planned social get-togethers, where everyone has fun—by learning to dance, of course—seniors are talked into signing expensive and binding contracts as high as $1,400. Some seniors have been known to go into a higher bracket: $5,000.

There are many senior citizen clubs, community recreation centers, libraries and YMCAs offering companionship and leisure activity to our older population. Usually the names are listed in your telephone directory or can be had by calling your city's information bureau.

Beware the work-at-home fraud! Now with the dollar's shrinking purchasing power, many seniors are feeling the pinch and are looking for ways to supplement their income. A few unscrupulous people advertise work-at-home employment such as knitting machine work, weaving or work on similar small equipment. The sponsoring firm agrees to purchase the finished articles "providing they meet certain standards," and that's the catch. After a few sales, your product is never going to be up to "certain standards." The company's only interest is selling the machine— not you and your financial status!

Many seniors, because they have time on their hands and the past is so vivid in their minds, decide to write. "My that's good! You should get it published!" well-meaning friends tell them. Suddenly, in their minds they see their name on a book, and with that, acclaim, fame, friends and fortune; they're not lonely any more.

One woman who wrote vividly of her early childhood put her life's savings, $10,000, into the publication of her book, which sold for $5 a copy. The first 100 copies went like wildfire to family and friends, and then the boom was over. She tried to get bookstores to market it for her (she couldn't get a distributor)—they took three on consignment. So, because it was her life savings, she decided to market them herself at fairs, antique shows, any place she could secure a free corner to display them. Three years later, she had recovered less than $3,000.

Seniors must be aware of investing their money in publishing ventures. All they are going to get is the satisfaction of seeing a book with their name on the cover. Any secret dreams of recovering the cost of publication and going on to fame and fortune, is just that—a secret dream.

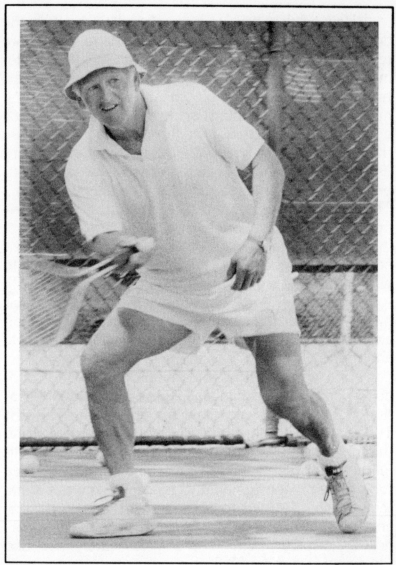

Lynda Middleton

Usually at Christmas your mailbox will be cram-
med with books, calendars, trinkets and other items
from firms who hope you will respond with a check.
Remember, you don't have to pay for unsolicited
merchandise that arrives by mail. And you don't have

to spend money on postage to return it. If you are badgered for payment, write to Consumer Advocate, U.S. Postal Service, Washington, D.C., 20260.

And there are the pressure salespersons who put their foot in the door, or who, once they are in, stay until two or three in the morning, just hammering away until you buy. Because seniors are tired and confused, they buy and the bill is often several hundred dollars. If a high-pressure salesperson gets in and you want him or her to leave but can't make them go, just call the police. If you do weaken and sign, the next morning get legal aid.

There are other crimes, other frauds that are more subtle, and because of their nature are not prosecutable. They usually involve family, close friends, down-and-outers who "just need a chance."

"Aunt Mae, now that Uncle Edward is gone, you won't be able to look after the farm—and you know my wife and family haven't been having it easy—so, if you'll sign the farm over to me, I'll look after it for you and see that you have a home for the rest of your life."

Mae signed over the farm, and she did have a home (an upstairs apartment was created for her) but as the years passed, the burden of her care became heavier, and the weight of her nephew's debt to her became lighter. Before Mae knew it, she was in a retirement home. She had sold a hundred-acre farm for seven years' care.

Older people are extremely vulnerable in today's fast-moving world of business. The old-fashioned way of doing business with a handshake and a my-word-is-my-bond contract is as outdated as the horse and buggy. The depth of the family circle has receded with the times. Yet one thing which was true then, is true today—we can save ourselves a lot of trouble by using common sense.

Transportation

Cars play a crucial role in the lives of seniors. For many, a car is the only way to go, the hub of their mobility. Seniors depend on their cars for shopping, medical appointments and recreation. For them, loss of wheels is catastrophic.

In the United States seniors make up 10% of the driving public, yet according to the 1977 statistics, they are involved in more accidents per mile than any group except teenagers.

Why is their record so bad? They rarely drive when road conditions are hazardous and they are more courteous—so where does the problem lie?

The University of Michigan's Institute of Gerontology decided to find out. After four years of study, using statistics from police departments, insurance companies and state transportation departments, they came to the conclusion that the high accident rate was simply due to the aging process.

Dr. Leon Pastalan, who supervised the study, says, "As people grow older there is a subtle but gradual decline in the sensitivity of their senses. Although they don't recognize it, seniors have normal losses in vision, hearing, smell and touch."

The remedy suggested by the study was not so simple. Seniors have to be made aware of the fact that they are now accident prone, and they have to learn to compensate for this decline in their senses.

Poor vision seems to be the main culprit in accidents involving older people. Minnie, for example, was a typical senior driver who until three months ago, when she ran into the rear end of another car, had never had an accident. Her problem—depth perception. Minnie had misjudged the distance between her car and the one ahead. "So how do I cope?" she wailed. The answer: a driver refresher course.

Minnie found that over a period of years a deterioration in her vision had crept up unnoticed. Her judgment of distance was not as accurate as it once was. And although she still had 20-20 vision, her reflexes had slowed.

If you want to make a simple test to see if age has affected your driving ability (our steering coordination peaks at 25), try backing into a regular uptown parking space or your own garage. Remember, this used to be done on the first try! How many times did it take now? One, two, three? Seniors must recognize their limitations; they must police themselves.

Many seniors refuse to believe they have changed with the years, that today is not yesterday. Joe believed he was as good as he ever was—until he got into an accident.

Joe lives on the outskirts of a small community. His nearest neighbor is a mile away. He depends on his car to get groceries, to take his wife to the doctor (she doesn't drive), to go to church and to take them to social outings. His car is a necessity.

Suddenly Joe's whole lifestyle changed: he lost his license. His accident was not a serious one, but it could have been! Joe pulled into a moving line of traffic and didn't properly gauge the speed of the on-coming car. In many areas any senior citizen involved in an accident must automatically take a driver's test. Joe failed his test.

Why? Not because he couldn't drive, but because he hadn't kept abreast of new road regulations. He was driving yesterday's way; he hadn't made allowances for changes in himself or in the times.

Many seniors started driving 40 to 50 years ago and their ability is based strictly on experience. Their knowledge and understanding of driving laws and driving procedures are out of date.

This was Edward's problem. He failed to yield the right of way. His idea of yielding and the law's defini-tion were totally different. He was charged.

In order to make sure he passed his driver's test, which was mandatory (Edward was 82), he enrolled in a privately-tutored course, and before the first lesson was finished, he was amazed at what he didn't know. Although he had taken note of the changing road signs over the years, he had never read any booklets on the new laws and regulations of the road.

"My first car was a 1926 Ford Speedster," he said. "I got my first driving lesson steering that Speedster up and down the back lane of Dad's farm—even the cows took off when they saw me coming."

Edward, before he took his refresher course, always believed slow driving and cautious driving were the same. His instructor said no! Slow drivers cause many accidents because they impede the speed of the driver behind them; the driver behind chomps on the bit and will often take unnecessary chances just to get by.

"If you notice a long line of traffic behind you, pull off the road, in a safe place of course, and let the traffic proceed. Before you pull out again, check and recheck to make sure you're clear," the instructor told him.

By the time Edward finished the eight-week course, he had regained his confidence and had decided to take a cross-country trip. He made his trip, and it went without a hitch. He took his time; he avoided night driving; he often took the secondary highways instead of the fast-moving expressways and throughways. He wasn't in any hurry. Time was on his side, and he made it work for him.

Dr. I C. Gryfe, medical director of Baycrest Centre for Geriatric Care, guest speaker at the annual meeting of the Ontario chapter of the College of Family Physicians of Canada, says, "A patient's medical history and not chronological age is the most important factor in judging fitness to drive."

Alertness at the wheel is a must. If you are on medication, check your reflexes. If they are dulled, don't drive. Take public transit or a taxi—they'll be cheaper in the long run.

Statistics show the main causes of accidents among senior citizens are inattention, failure to signal, failure to observe stop signs, and unreasonably slow driving. Another rule to adhere to is "if you've had a few, don't drive!" Dr. Gryfe says, "Alcoholism causes greater impairment of reflex action than celebrating one's 90th birthday."

Sam McLeod/The London Free Press

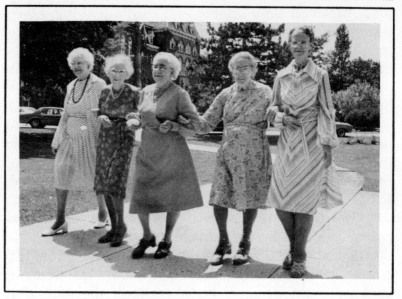

Often, cars, like the seniors who drive them, are getting older; they too need safety checks. Make sure windows and headlights are clean. Seniors need all the advantages they can get.

Drive defensively! This means recognizing hazards, looking well ahead, even at the car in front of the car ahead of you—getting the overall picture. It means knowing how to drive in adverse weather conditions and compensating for them. It means looking out for the other guy—he may be a nut!

It's a wise person who looks both ways before proceeding through a green light, and another defensive measure worth remembering—pick a point ahead, even with the lead car, then if you arrive at that point in less than two seconds, you are following too closely. In bad weather, it's wise to keep one-tenth of a mile behind the vehicle in front of you. Never, never drive with the wolfpack!

Cars add a great deal to the quality of life for senior citizens, although now with the rising cost of gasoline, we must reassess their value. A few insurance companies are raising their rates at age 65, but most, as long as a senior has a valid license, are willing to take the risk at no additional cost, although some ask for a simple medical certificate for those 70 and over.

Although many drive, some seniors over-depend on others to take them places. How often have you heard, "I'll go if someone will take me"? Rarely do these people ever compensate the driver.

Alternatives are now being offered, and even if you still drive, it's wise to be aware of them, because there might be a time in the future when you can't drive.

Dial-a-bus is available in many communities, and is usually sponsored by a service club, thus keeping costs to a minimum. Public transit is available in all major cities, and if you must take a taxi, why not try pooling the costs with two or three other seniors? And there is nothing wrong with walking; it is the cheapest exercise you can find.

One community has a determined alderman who has come up with an idea which is helping a number of seniors with their shopping.

William McCulloch, in cooperation with Dominion Stores, has put a plan into operation that costs the taxpayer nothing, yet provides a convenient shopping service for seniors. The plan, now in its third year, is working so successfully that other communities are modeling their proposed "service for seniors" after it.

"A project of this type can only work in a high-density area," McCulloch stresses, "and then we are only able to go out every two weeks."

His plan is simple: a bus rented from a local line comes to a designated location, picks up a group of seniors and takes them to a local Dominion Store. The bus then leaves for another location, with Alderman

103

McCulloch usually in attendance, where they pick up 40-47 more seniors and return to the store, where the first load of shoppers is waiting to be taken home.

"Since we run on a very tight schedule, we can't wait for anyone, but the seniors police themselves," he said. He tries to keep the bus rental costs to a minimum with a maximum rental time of two hours. "This way we can break even."

The whole operation costs out at 50 cents per person, which is split equally between the senior citizen and Dominion Stores. "We do have bus tickets, but not the regular ones; this is so we can control the number using the service. We can't have 60 seniors scheduled for one run with only 47 seats on the bus."

It was the store's decision to choose Wednesday afternoon as the best time for the seniors to visit, mainly because it is their slow time, and the weekend specials are available. The store, which has extra staff on during these two hours, caters to seniors' needs by packaging smaller portions of meats and vegetables. "There are many older people who find a head of cabbage just too much for them," said a produce clerk. "With so many seniors shopping at one time we can cut a cabbage or lettuce in half without fear of wasting the other half."

Senior citizen volunteers are also at the store and at the drop-off points to assist those who need help with their packages. These volunteers are assisted by students from local high schools who are involved in the community work program. The students push the carts and carry out the bags of groceries. "They enjoy the privilege of getting out of school for a couple of hours, and they also enjoy swapping stories with the older people," Alderman McCulloch said.

He also feels that a shopping tour like this would not work successfully every week because seniors just

104

don't buy that many groceries, and there is a cost factor for the store. A shopper must spend about $10 if the store's participation in paying half the cost per person for the bus rental is to be really worth the expense.

In the relatively short time this service has been in operation, McCulloch estimates they have taken more than 10,000 seniors shopping. "People working with the seniors tell me they are eating better, using more fresh fruits and vegetables."

This bus shuttle has become an important alternative in the lives of these seniors. Thanks to a little bit of ingenuity and some horse sense, it is working, and there isn't any reason why it couldn't work in other communities. It just needs someone with drive, like William McCulloch, to put it into operation.

Some of this same drive is needed in rural communities where seniors suffer most when wheels are lost. Why is it not feasible for two or three counties to pool their resources, get a small bus, hire a driver and once every two weeks set up a route to take seniors in a particular area shopping or to the doctor? This way, if these older citizens were sure of a ride, they could arrange their appointments and style of living accordingly. The same bus and the same driver would service another area the next day, and so on. Since the cost would be split between the counties participating, it would not be that great. Seniors should not receive this service free; they should be charged a fee in keeping with income. In this age of pensions and supplements, seniors don't need to be free-loaders. Free-loading is demeaning.

It is true cars add much to the quality of life of our seniors, but now with costs escalating, we must question their value. There are alternatives; explore them in your area—there could be a better way to travel.

Owning Your Home

"To be happy at home is the ultimate aim of all ambition; the end to which every enterprise and labor tends."—Samuel Johnson.

People nowadays feel the same way Dr. Johnson did 200 years ago, but their ambition to own their own home is being thwarted by inflation, taxes and high repair costs. Many who have struggled for years to make mortgage payments now find that even though their property is clear of debt, they can no longer afford to stay in their own homes.

Yet one of the most important aspects of retirement is a senior's accommodation—wherever you live, your surroundings and the kind of housing you have will directly affect the quality of your life.

Aware of the social, psychological and economic importance of seniors remaining in their own homes, boards of health, national senior councils and many other arms of government are recommending that older people be given greater tax credits, while those who rent should be given supplements to encourage them to stay out of institutions.

Actually, when seniors retire, they have four courses open to them: stay where they are, sell their big home and buy a smaller one, sell and then rent an apartment or smaller home, or lease their big home and use the revenue to rent a smaller place.

Statistics show that in the United States almost 70% of those 65 and over prefer to stay put; another 25% do move but remain in the general area; only 5% move completely away. A warm climate may look very inviting in the winter, but it is a different story in the summer. There is no such thing as a perfect climate in which to retire, despite the growing popularity of retirement areas in Arizona and Florida.

By the time seniors reach retirement age, their homes are usually paid for but in need of extensive repair. For instance, the life of a roof is about twenty years, and by that time, plumbing and wiring will also need fixing. With only their pensions and a small inflation-eroded savings account, seniors haven't got the money to cope with costly improvements.

Before you definitely decide to sell, there are some things you had better check. How much does it cost you to live in your present home? Add up the amounts you pay each year for taxes, fuel, insurance, utilities, repairs, etc., and divide by 12. Could you live as happily and cheaply anywhere else?

If you invested your money from the sale of your house, would it cover rental costs? If not, you are farther ahead to stay where you are. If your home is large, you might decide to rent it and move to smaller quarters: would the rent or lease money cover the large home's expenses and your new ones? Remember, you would still be responsible for maintenance of the old home, and if there is profit in such an undertaking, don't forget, it's taxable.

Before you decide to do anything, look into the

options available to you. Some "band-aid" assistance now comes in the form of municipal rebates on education taxes, but there is a catch—if a retiree's house is sold, the rebate is reclaimed by the municipality. Ask about the rebate at your local city hall; it may apply in your area.

The Ontario Home Renewal Program gave band-aid relief when it came up with the idea that anyone whose income was less than $12,500 could receive assistance with repair costs. Part of the cost, up to $4,000, would be an outright grant, and the rest would be in the form of a loan repayable at an adjusted-to-income rate of interest.

For those seniors who have been in the service, different veteran organizations offer assistance for home repairs for veterans and their families. Although most local branches can only assist in minor areas, the parent organization such as the Canadian Legion in Canada have money available, or can obtain it through the Federal Department of Veteran's Affairs.

One large city has a new program that provides high school students to help clean and maintain seniors' homes; if necessary, they will also assist with the shopping. Many programs like this have been started across North America, but many of them are short-lived. About six or seven months after their demise, a similar program starts, and the same ground must be covered at extra expense; by the time seniors are aware of "help to stay in their homes" programs, the help has often gone down the proverbial drain.

Seniors, unable to see to their own repairs, are often fair game for con artists who like to prey on older citizens, especially widows.

At 68, Mrs. S. found herself responsible for paying bills and looking after repairs, jobs her husband had done for the last 41 years. When a man wearing a coverall uniform with an insignia over the breastpocket knocked on her door and said, "I'm from the . . . mumble . . . agency; I've come to inspect your furnace," she let him in, even though she wasn't having any furnace problems.

A few minutes later the man came up from the basement. "It's in bad shape!" he said. "Don't know how it has lasted this long." He had two rusted parts in his hand. "There's no sense in putting it back together—just a waste of time." He left.

So now Mrs. S. not only had a furnace that was in bad shape, she also had one that was in several pieces. Then, unexpectedly, an excellent furnace repairman came to the door. He had heard from the "agency" man that Mrs. S. was having problems. He had a mother living on the east coast; Mrs. S. reminded him of her; he hoped someone would look after her interests while he was working in Tonawanda.

Then the furnace man gave Mrs. S. an estimate.

"That's an awful lot of money!" she gasped. Her husband had left her comfortably fixed, but with inflation, her savings were shrinking faster than she had anticipated. Regardless, she had to have heat, so she ordered a new furnace.

Several weeks later, on one of the coldest nights in January, her furnace broke down again. She tried to contact the furnace man. He wasn't listed in the Yellow Pages—in fact, he wasn't listed anywhere. In desperation, she called another heating company. They sent their man; he inspected the furnace. "I'm afraid you need a whole new unit."

"That's impossible," she cried. "That one was new three months ago." She hunted up her canceled check; she had never received a receipt.

Like so many others, Mrs. S. had been conned, and it was all done by "such a nice man." Some seniors still believe business is done today as it was in the 1920s, when one's word was one's bond and a handshake sealed every agreement. Today everything must be put into writing, *especially estimates*, and seniors are advised to get not just one, but two or three.

Seniors are at their most vulnerable when dealing with crafts and repair people. Many of the builders, carpenters, electricians and plumbers they have known through the years have, like themselves, grown older; many have retired. A new generation is in business.

David R. bought his house shortly after he returned from overseas in 1946. He and his wife scrimped to make the payments and in 1971 the final payment was made. That house is now 33 years old, and many things are going wrong.

Three years ago David suffered a stroke that left his left arm and right leg nearly useless. Last year his wife died, but in spite of everything, David is determined to stay in his own home, and with the help of the Red Cross Homemaker Service, he is doing just that. His biggest problems are getting the lawn mowed in summer, the windows washed on the outside and having the eavestroughs cleaned.

David is a perfectionist. He likes everything done at the moment it needs doing. For weeks last spring he had been after his son to clean the windows, but his son had a home of his own and a young family and his time was limited.

An ad appeared in the local paper in early May. "Young man will clean windows, $8 an hour." David thought the rate high, but he needed the work done.

He called the number; the man said he would come the next day. Instead of one, two came; the window cleaner and a helper to handle the extension ladder. When David received his bill four hours later, it totaled $96.

He was flabbergasted. They had cleaned four regular-size and one small kitchen window, one picture window and two smaller upstairs ones. "How did you arrive at this figure?" David demanded.

It was simple arithmetic: the hourly rate for four hours for two men, plus traveling time and rental of the ladder. David paid. He didn't want anyone to know about his being "taken" because his two sons had been trying to persuade him to go to a home for the aged; this incident would give them added ammunition.

To deal with the need of seniors for reliable repair people, a few communities have organized "skills banks" of retired tradesmen who still want to keep a little active. When a senior needs service, they call the bank.

Some of these retired and semi-retired people may move a shade slower, but their work is of the highest quality. They learned their trades when pride in one's work was valued more highly than the money stuffed into a pay envelope.

In Great Britain the Link Skills Exchange Centres have become highly successful. Based on the barter system (instead of trading goods, they trade skills) it has saved seniors thousands of pounds. It is an inexpensive set-up—there's no red tape, no paid staff. The coordinating center is manned by people who receive a barter token or stamp for each hour worked. Because no money is exchanged, the income and benefits of either the giver or the receiver are not affected.

The system works this way: Mrs. Lawson needs her ironing board fixed. She phones the local Link Exchange Services and is put in touch with Ray Watts. He repairs her ironing board and she pays him in Link tokens or stamps. He adds these to others he has earned and gives them to Mattie Hornblower who mends his socks and sews buttons on his shirt. Mrs.

111

Hornblower, in turn, uses her stamps or tokens to pay for music lessons from a retired teacher, and so the system goes, helping seniors stay in their own homes.

There are many different types of housing for seniors to choose from: independent units, which includes single family homes in communities and retirement villages, second homes, which includes vacation and mobile homes, and multi-units, which takes in condominiums, apartments and cooperatives.

Mobile homes, because of their low cost, are very popular in the United States; one out of every ten retirees lives in a mobile home. Financing is available, with as little as 5% down and 15 years to pay, but one fact that seniors must keep in mind is that these mobiles depreciate faster than a standard house.

Hundreds of multi-unit dwellings are now being built in North America, and for seniors seeking freedom from gardening and other chores, these are the answer. They are usually close to public transportation, shopping centers, medical offices and churches. About one out of every eight apartments is now a cooperative or condominium. The main difference between these two is that condominium owners hold the title on their individual units, while cooperatives are owned by stockholders, the occupant being a stockholder. There is also more freedom in selling a condominium—it is yours to do with as you please—but in the sale of a cooperative, other shareholders must be consulted and the new buyer approved.

In these multi-unit dwellings, no one is segregated. People with children, seniors, handicapped, all live side by side, and each family contributes to the community, especially in the cooperatives, where everyone helps everyone else.

One theory that has been put into practice in a few scattered areas is "double up and save money."

Seniors with large homes and lots of empty rooms turn them into sanctuaries for others.

Each couple has a separate bedroom, sitting room and sometimes a bath. They share a common kitchen, living room and dining area. However, this practice has been severely curtailed because zoning regulations in many areas state that one-family homes can't be turned into two- or three-family dwellings, even though the owner and tenants share cost of fuel, electricity and taxes. But the energy crisis has caused us to take a hard look at our lifestyles. What better way to conserve energy than to have five or six seniors sharing the same refrigerator and dishwasher, and eating under the same electric lights?

Share-a-home is not a new concept; it has been working in Florida for some years. Share-a-home works on the same premise as the old-fashioned boardinghouse or tourist home, except that the members of the household run their home as equal members of a family.

Some communities have carried share-a-home a step further: they provide a resident manager. He and his wife will provide guidance and counselling and look after recreation and transportation needs.

Another idea has found merit: taking old school buildings out of retirement. The buildings are paid for, they usually have a good-size yard, and they stand empty and forlorn. Why not recycle them into senior citizen housing? Input from older people themselves is needed; if seniors don't speak up and make their needs known, how are others going to know exactly what they want?

Granny flats have been the answer for many seniors in the Australian state of Victoria. They are self-contained, single-storey dwellings with floor space of approximately 378 square feet, designed for easy installation in an average-size Australian suburban backyard.

The first granny flat was built in 1975 by the Victoria Housing Commission from an idea presented by the Victoria Council of the Aged. The flats have a timber floor and modular timber-frame walls, and come complete with plumbing, electrical fittings, floor coverings and complete interior decoration. When flats become vacant through death or for other reasons, they can be easily dismantled and rebuilt elsewhere.

There are several designs for seniors to choose from: smaller single units renting at $15 a month, and large "couple" units at $20. All contain a bedroom, bathroom-toilet and living room with kitchen annex.

These granny flats enable older people to maintain their independence and still be near their families, in fact, in their backyard, but the tensions which build up from having different age groups living in the same house are nullified. This same idea could be adapted to any community with sufficient yard space. It's certainly worth investigating.

Seniors need to live in their own homes as long as possible; it is not only their right, it is for their own good. To live happily among furnishings that are familiar, to be able to touch old memories, can be far more crucial to a senior's well-being than excellent care at a big, anonymous institution. Home is where the heart is—and a senior's heart is in his or her own home.

Senior Citizen Housing

During the last decade high-rise complexes have become a way of life for thousands and thousands of seniors. Since most of these units have rents in direct ratio to income, almost every segment of the senior population can afford them.

However, there is more to unit-living than just moving in, and many seniors are finding it difficult to adjust to this mode of accommodation, especially those who have lived in rural towns and villages.

Looking down the 200-foot-long corridor with closed doors every 20 feet, one senior said, "It is just like a cell, only I have the key." He had spent most of his life on the family farm.

His neighbor Joe loved his bachelor apartment. He could afford it, and it was easy to keep clean. "Let's face it, the next move for me will be into a nursing home, so I'm going to enjoy my independence as long as I can."

The main difference between the two men was the attitude they brought with them. Joe had come by choice. Arthur had come by necessity. His big rambling house had been too much for him, both physically and financially.

Senior apartments provide an answer to the housing needs of pensioners and those with small savings, but the loneliness in some of these cracker boxes is overwhelming. Less than 35% of the tenants in high-rise complexes take part in the goings-on of the building. Another 30% will take part in the odd activity, the rest will remain behind closed doors.

Rev. Bruce Pocock has worked for five years in community relations and family services. He feels one of the greatest needs in these high-rises is tenant associations. "They should not be just bitch associations," he says, "they should be involved with the leisure activity needs of the people in that particular building."

Usually when seniors move into a high-rise, they have sold their homes, and at this point in their lives are wholly dependent on their landlord, often a large government agency.

Often, when they are having a problem, they need someone to speak for them; they are no longer capable of standing up and shouting on their own behalf. Tenant associations can make their needs known.

Unfortunately, in many ways senior citizen housing rests under the wing of all levels of government and is therefore susceptible to political logic and to budgets based on raising the least trouble with voters. Since cost is always a guiding factor, the best sites are not always chosen. A board, usually with no senior citizen representation, decides what is best for those on the senior side. Sometimes these giant complexes are built in low-lying areas, on secondary roads, away from the main stream of traffic. Seniors rely heavily on public transportation, and location can be a problem if the transportation system closes down certain routes at seven or eight at night.

"The people who designed these complexes certainly never had to live in them, nor were they ever in the moving business," said a tenant. Before becoming a resident, he had been associated with a moving and storage company.

Moving seniors into high-rises can be a nightmare for the movers, especially when they have two customers moving in on the same day, on the same floor, and there is a difference of over a hundred dollars in the two bills.

"Just try to satisfactorily explain to Mrs. L. that her apartment was at the opposite end of the corridor, the farthest possible point from the elevator," said the dispatcher. "Mrs. R.'s apartment was twelve feet from the elevator, and she had just a few cartons, while Mrs. L. had dozens."

Although rates vary, most moving companies have an hourly rate plus a surcharge for high-rise movings. When moving long distances, shipments are charged on the weight system; in most cities, there is another surcharge for the core areas.

Sometimes, when one has a family, it is cheaper to do it yourself, although sometimes the saving doesn't offset the frustrations.

When Sybil decided to move to a high-rise, her family was quite pleased; her six-room, storey-and-a-half house was just too much for her. The apartment sounded wonderful—until her problems started.

Sybil had a dog. He too was old, and since the senior citizen housing would not allow pets, she had to have him put to sleep. To her it was like having a friend put to death.

For weeks after the final agreement of sale was signed, she would spend one day sorting and discarding the treasures of a lifetime of living, and the next day she would reclaim all the pieces that she just couldn't part with. Finally her son told her, "An auc-

117

tioneer is coming over to have a look at the appliances and upstairs furniture."

Sybil cried when the man left. She had never realized her things were in such terrible condition. The auctioneer had offered her $400 for the lot, and he would remove them the afternoon of moving day.

"You had better book your mover ahead," a neighbor advised. "They get busy towards the end of the month, and you're moving the last day of March."

Sybil chose the company recommended by the butcher on the corner. When she called, the dispatcher said they could have a truck there at 8 a.m. on the morning of the 31st. Happy now that everything was set, she called her son who lived in a nearby village.

"How much are they charging you?" he asked.

"Thirty-five dollars an hour for a truck and two men," she answered.

"That's highway robbery!" he exclaimed. "I can get a buddy of mine who has a feed truck, and we'll move you for one quarter of that price."

Money was a definite concern, so Sybil canceled the movers. Three days before she was to take possession of her apartment her son called. His buddy couldn't get the truck. His advice, call the movers back.

Reluctantly Sybil called the company with whom she had originally booked. "I'm sorry, madam, we're booked solid!" Sybil called the other three movers in her town; their response was the same.

Then a few hours later, the family to whom she had sold the house, called. "Our furniture will arrive by 10 a.m. on the 31st."

Frustrated, upset, confused, Sybil called her son. He became angry. Why should he assume all the responsibility? She had two daughters!

Not knowing where to turn, Sybil started to cry.

Her moving had suddenly become a nightmare. In desperation she called her daughter in Fredericton. She was just leaving for a vacation in Florida. Sybil called her other daughter in Montreal: "I'll be there as soon as I can get a flight," her younger daughter said.

At first she didn't have any more luck getting a mover than Sybil. Finally one mover called back; he had had a cancellation at two o'clock on the 31st. Although it wasn't early enough, she didn't hesitate: "Book it!"

The people who had bought the house were very unhappy when they arrived and found that Sybil was still there, and they told her so in no uncertain terms. However, by four in the afternoon she was in her new apartment, the furniture was in place, her clothes were in the closet, and one of the most trying experiences in her life was over.

She didn't know until later that had her movers been running behind schedule, the caretaker would not have allowed her to move into her high-rise apartment that day—all movings in or out had to be done between 9:00 and 5:00, and this time restriction was strictly enforced.

Sybil was soon to learn a few more things about apartment living that she didn't know or suspect. The caretaker in her senior citizen high-rise was a little dictator who had a phobia about having the cleanest building in the city. During his younger years he had been a sergeant-major in the army, and now he observed the spit-and-polish of the army barracks.

Sybil, like most seniors, took good care of her apartment; she respected the landlord's property and was a good tenant in every way. In her particular building, each tenant had to take the garbage to a special bin at the back entrance. One day, on her way there, the bag split (she "hadn't been listening to the

119

right commercials") and some strawberry juice was spilled on the carpet. Instead of helping her clean it up, the caretaker ranted and raved until he had Sybil in tears. She was so upset that any garbage she had after that she packaged into her shopping bag and took to a friend's house, where she set it at the curb for the garbageman.

After the strawberry juice episode Sybil kept more and more to her apartment; and when she had to go out, she darted in and out like a frightened rabbit. She became jumpy and edgy and everything worried her; in fact, she worried herself into the hospital with a nervous condition.

Not all caretakers are like the one in Sybil's building; some take their jobs of helping the tenants very seriously and the seniors love them. However, it is always the bad apples we hear about and not the good ones.

Housing administrators are now becoming aware that the janitorial staff should receive training. They have to be able to accept complaints and problems— the tenants are not there for the caretaker's benefit, he is there for theirs. Harassment of tenants is becoming too common and if a senior feels compelled to move— so what? There are a dozen others waiting to take the unit.

"At our complex we have a beautiful lawn and several plots of flowers. One day I walked across the lawn and picked a rose," a senior said. She was speaking at an inquiry hearing into senior housing. "Before I even straightened up, the building custodian was yelling and frantically waving his arms, 'Get off the lawn! Your heels are digging into my grass!' (She was wearing a pair of wedge sandals at the time.) 'And you can't pick them flowers; they're for show!'"

Unfortunately, many custodians see their build-

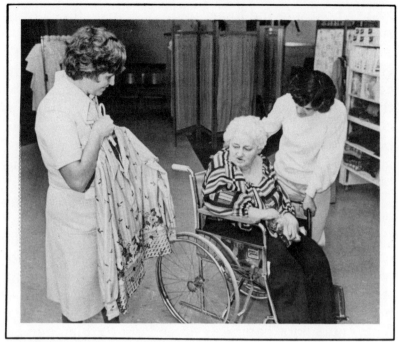

Ed Heal/The London Free Press

ings as a "show." They turn their complexes into clean, sterile edifices where seniors can come and go, but not use and enjoy.

At the same hearing, an 83-year-old tenant from a neighboring building, who is crippled with arthritis, told the committee, "As soon as I opened the front door, he was shouting, 'Take off your boots! You've got snow on your feet!'"

She went on to say that the reason she wore her boots into and out of the building was that it took her 20 minutes to get them off and on, an act she performed inside her apartment. She wasn't going to allow others to watch her. She didn't want pity.

After one incident in a high-rise out west came to light, a caretaker got the axe. In that particular building, seniors mingled well and once a month had a dance. Unfortunately, because of lack of space, they

121

had to hold it in the foyer, with, of course, the permission of the housing authority.

So that their steps would slip and slide a little easier, they sprinkled dance wax on the floor. As the couples laughed and danced, they were interrupted by the caretaker with his mop and bucket, swishing his cleaning mixture over the floor. When they complained, he answered, "No one is going to say I neglected my duties. Slippery floors are a no-no in this building!"

And at the hearing, someone told about a woman who was so intimidated by the man in charge of her building that when a fuse blew in her stove and she couldn't locate it, she went without hot food for almost three weeks until her son came to visit and fix it. By this time the woman's health had deteriorated—it took several days at his house to get her back on her feet. This senior had been singled out for blame many times by the caretaker because the rubber tip of her cane occasionally scuffed his floor. Seniors, especially women who have been used to having a husband stick up for them, are especially vulnerable to this kind of harassment.

At the hearing another man told the committee, "One of the things we miss is the children. At our pre-retirement residence, all generations were mixed together. We feel the pendulum has swung too greatly in preference to seniors—now we are being ostracized."

Senior citizen housing, whether high-rise or town house, is a blessing. It has solved many needs, but the buildings themselves cannot solve the loneliness or the fear, only people can do that. Until planners, developers, architects and administrators truly feel the needs of the older population, many unnecessary problems will continue to exist.

Nursing Homes and Homes for the Aged

There are basically two types of institutions for the elderly: nursing homes, which are privately owned, and homes for the aged, which are owned by a municipal or regional government, with the average age of residents being 82.

Great strides have been made to bring both types of institution out of the 19th century and get them ready for the 21st. Nursing homes and homes for the aged have come a long way in improving their image, yet they still have a long way to go. Although many resemble glorified hotels, the stigma of the "old folks home" still clings.

Nursing homes are being upgraded; care is being improved; environment, too, is being taken into consideration. It's a whole new ball game.

Along with this improvement in institutionalized care, gerontology itself is coming of age. Now people who work with the elderly are being recognized as specialists in their field. Too often in the past, a person only accepted a position in care-for-the-elderly institutions when there was nothing else available; geriatric care was considered the bottom of the ladder. Thank goodness, this is beginning to change. In 1975 the Gerontological Nursing Association was founded, primarily to help focus attention on geriatrics as a creative specialty within the nursing profession.

Dr. Gustave Gingras, a director of rehabilitation services for a regional department of health, said in a recent speech, "Teachers of medical and health sciences are youth-oriented. For too many, the common problems of the aged are less interesting than those more dramatic ailments to younger persons—as the dramatic effect fades, so does the interest."

So important is this new image that one nursing home association has promoted dozens of regional workshops over the last two years, which not only deal with the basic problems of putting tired old bodies back into motion, but also with the whole person.

"A home for the aged must be an integral part of the community, and the community must be a part of the home," says Fred Boyse, administrator of Elgin Manor and Terrace Lodge, two well-known homes for the aged.

Terrace Lodge, built in 1976, has many unique features, and is considered to be one of the finest and most progressive homes for the aged in North America. Couples have scaled-down apartments furnished with pieces of their own furniture; the lodge has its own post office and residents have their own box and key. Residents can also make use of a snack shop, beauty parlor, barber shop and "quiet room," all deliberately placed at the front of the building so that they will have to leave their rooms if they want anything.

"We feel this encourages residents to get out and mingle, rather than retreat," Fred says.

The idea of Terrace Lodge was first outlined on

the back of a restaurant menu while he was having dinner with two friends. In one year he spoke to more than 150 groups and clubs, describing his plans. In return, he received over $42,000 in donations for extra equipment and furnishings.

Terrace Lodge has a swimming pool (the water temperature is kept at 80 degrees) and a bowling alley, as well as spacious lawns.

If more homes for the aged of the high caliber of Terrace Lodge are to be built, seniors themselves must get involved—few communities have dedicated men like Fred Boyse. Doors need to be opened; architects, city planners and developers must be made more aware of the ideas and concerns of the elderly, and these can only come from them. They are the ones most qualified to know.

Nursing homes are run for people and for profit, but too often dollars and cents are the prime motivating factor. The help may leave a lot to be desired because help is hard to get—in some homes the staff turnover is as high as 50% and because of the great need, there is only token training.

This is one of the areas where resident councils can help. They can be the bridge between the administration and the patients.

A resident council is a group of residents in a nursing home or home for the aged working together, using democratic principles for the common good within the institution. Resident councils aren't meant to manage; they guide, gathering opinions, ideas and complaints. They work much like a municipal council, with their own rules, procedures and agendas, but they must provide much more than lip service if they are going to be effective.

A resident councilor must be a listener as well as an observer. "Who is going to listen to some old woman's complaints?'' said one aide, taunting a patient who threatened to go to the administrator. The aide was right—no one would listen; there was no resident council in operation in that home.

One of the main advantages of having a resident council is that there is always someone who will listen. When a patient has a complaint, he or she can take it to the council member, who will take it to the mayor. Nor does it have to be the patient—a friend, relative or roommate who sees a problem can report it. If the complaint is legitimate, the council will take it to the administration.

The administrator, after checking thoroughly into the matter, which in the case of the "old woman" was undue cruelty on the part of an attendant giving an enema, took corrective steps; the attendant was dismissed.

Both homes for the aged and, to a lesser degree, nursing homes still have to fight the stigma of the past, not many years ago, when elderly people, the aunts, uncles, and sometimes the mothers and fathers of today's retirees, were committed to old age homes.

In these archaic institutions seniors had to work as much as they could for their keep; men and women were separated and visiting was restricted. Many homes allowed no visitors on Sundays, except clergy. These homes didn't just put seniors to death swiftly, as our primitive ancestors did, they buried them alive for endless years in jails from which there was only one escape.

Although supportive services are doing much to keep seniors in their own homes, sometimes institutional care cannot be avoided. Health deteriorates, memory slows, legs become unsteady, and it is in the best interest of a senior to be admitted to a home. However, only a small percentage (4% or less) will have institutional care. There is a high death rate (30 to 50%) among the elderly who are waiting for admission, or who have just been admitted.

In spite of the growing integration between community and institution, there is still the fear, the utter dread, of being admitted to one. "You only come out one way—flat out!" one man said. In a way he was right. Few leave nursing homes to resume a normal life. "These places are like holding tanks where you wait for death."

Programs now are being tried to take some of the sting out of admission. Seniors Participate in Organized Recreation Therapy (SPORT), for example, is a program in which a local nursing home invites area seniors to share their facilities. Seniors, in turn, take residents on bus trips, theater outings and other recreational activities that include picnics and dancing. Through this gradual integration, it is hoped the transition from community to nursing home will be less traumatic.

How does one select the right nursing home or home for the aged? If you have a choice (sometimes there is none) what do you look for in way of accommodation, care and attitude of staff?

Angie found herself in the position of helping her father find an institution to which he could relocate without too much trauma. He was 80. He lived alone quite successfully for 10 years, then last year he tripped and fell on a turned-up corner of linoleum and broke his hip. A month ago he drifted off to sleep while watching TV. There was a small fire, which could have been serious, had not the paper boy smelled smoke and turned in an alarm. Yesterday, Henry forgot he had taken his pills and took them twice—he became ill and confused.

Like so many people, Angie didn't know where to

start looking for a suitable place for her father. Finally she got the telephone directory and began calling nursing homes.

"Sorry, we have a waiting list of more than 40," one administrator told her. Although her part of the country has over 450 licensed nursing homes, she soon found accommodation at a premium.

"Why don't you contact one of the homes for the aged?" one clerk asked, after Angie had explained her problem.

"I don't want to put my father in an old age home!" Angie cried. "Why, he would have to sign over everything he has to them!"

The admission clerk laughed. "I'm afraid you've been given a lot of wrong information," he said. He went on to say that since Henry, Angie's father, was not chronically ill, and he had lived more than a year in the county, he would be eligible for care, but probably they had a waiting list too.

Reluctantly, Angie called the home for the aged. No, she was told, they did not take the resident's money, although each applicant did have to report total assets.

"My father is quite able to pay his own way," Angie said. Her father had been a successful business-man and he still had a sizable bank account, plus his own home.

"He would still have to report his assets," the clerk answered. "However, this is confidential infor- mation and is kept locked in our files." She went on to explain that some people have only limited funds, and when those funds get to a low of $1,000, their account is picked up by the government.

"What about his pension?" Angie asked.

"Since your father is able to look after his own affairs, he will continue to do so," was the answer.

Each patient who paid his own way received a statement once a month. For those on a government pension, a portion of that pension called comfort allowance was returned to be used for clothing, recreation, pin money, or anything they might need.

"Father will be able to pay his own way, so will he receive better care, better facilities, better food?"

The clerk told her this wasn't the case. Every resident at a home for the aged receives the same care, and unless patients reveal the information, no one knows whether or not they pay their own way.

In her search for an answer to what to do with her father, Angie found that not all nursing homes or homes for the aged are the same. In some nursing homes where couples are admitted, husbands and wives are separated. Some homes like to keep their residents in bed attire, even during the day. Others encourage residents, if at all possible, to get up and dress. Although fire regulations have to be up to a certain standard, some homes have better fire escape facilities than others.

Angie learned that the attitude of staff toward patients differed too. In some homes everyone is called by his or her first name. In another Angie visited, only last names are used. She overheard one old gentleman, when he was called by his last name, reprimand a staff member by saying, "What's the matter, isn't the day long enough to call me mister?"

In another institution, restraints were used on many patients and drugs were used to control behavior. She read a report that said some gerontologists feel that the geriatric chair, with its small table attached to the front, is a restraint. Residents are helped into these chairs and left for hours on end with only a blank wall to look at. Angie checked on the use of this restraint chair.

129

She learned from a nurse about a man being "overprotected" by these restraints. After his problem came to light, the institution had modified its policy.

"This old fellow was always grumpy and morose; in fact, he was just plain miserable, but for the longest time no one tried to find out why. Then he got a new roommate who had a great deal of time to observe 'The Old Reprobate,' as he had been dubbed.

"Why don't you take off those restraints and just let him sit in a chair?" the roommate asked.

"Because he would have to be watched and we haven't got the time," the nurse's aide told him.

"Well, if you put him into a chair, I'll watch him," the roommate said.

Reluctantly, after more prodding, The Old Reprobate was put into a chair, and he began to perk up a little, but his eyes seemed heavy. Out of curiosity, the roommate counted the pills the old fellow had to take. "Can't you ease up on his medication a bit?" he asked.

"Doctor's orders!" the nurse snapped. She did not like interference from the patients.

Being a persistent cuss, the roommate took it upon himself to ask The Old Reprobate's doctor about the pills. The doctor listened sympathetically, and after consultation with the head nurse, reduced the medication.

Little by little The Old Reprobate came back into the world of the living; his senses became more in tune with his surroundings. The nurses could see an improvement, especially in his disposition, and they informed the doctor, who cut the medication even more and removed all restraints.

Less than a year later The Old Reprobate was walking around using a cane for support. He laughed and joked with fellow residents. He was alive again, all because one man cared. Now he is a member of that home's resident council.

Also in her search for a home for her father, Angie learned that day care service is offered as an alternative to full-time residency. Usually available on a five-day-week basis (anyone can register for a day at a time), seniors receive a hot noon meal or lunch, programs to improve their well-being, crafts training and use of recreational facilities, plus a chance to be with people their own age. For seniors who are constantly alone or who need some supervision in the daytime, day care is the answer.

Maxine is a teacher. She lives with her 83-year-old father, and although his health is good, he has a knee problem and can easily fall. When he falls he can't get up without assistance.

"We don't need a housekeeper," she says, "I can manage the work, but Dad just can't be left on his own all day."

With this new service available, Maxine can now drop her father off at the day care center in the home for the aged on her way to work; on her return in the afternoon she picks him up. Her father is happier too—he isn't alone so much. He's meeting people, doing craftwork and participating in current events discussions, which he loves.

For seniors on medication, staff members will make sure the pill or tonic is taken, although they usually will not be responsible for administering it.

Vacation care is another extension service. There are times when seniors need a vacation from the family, and the family needs a vacation from them. This government program allows individuals to apply to residence in a home for a temporary period, as long as there is room available. Most vacation care periods are about two or three weeks, but sometimes, under certain circumstances, they can be extended to a month.

Medication for vacation care residents is usually included in their care cost. Like other residents of a home, they must share a room. They are free to come and go as they please, the same as permanent residents. All the home's facilities such as swimming pool, craft shop and game room are available to them. Vacation care, a temporary residency, is also helpful for seniors who may sometime in the future become full-time residents; their stay gives them some idea of institutional living.

During her search, Angie had a great many feelings of guilt. When she got them into proper perspective, and after a consultation with her doctor, she took Henry to see both a nursing home and a home for the aged. It was a traumatic experience for him, but it was made a little easier when he discovered an old friend at one of the homes.

Not all seniors are as fortunate as Henry, who chose his residence. Many are committed by desperate relatives who must take the first bed available because they are at such a premium, and who are often not concerned about whether the new resident has semi-private or ward accommodation, just as long as it is a bed.

"Yet loss of privacy is one of the hardest parts of being institutionalized," says Patricia Kinsella, R.N., an executive board member of the Ontario Psychogeriatric Association. "Often the only thing between you and your neighbor is a half-drawn curtain."

It is very difficult for people who have been used to their own home to function in a four-bed room. These rooms have the beds placed with their heads against the side walls, with only a narrow passageway between. A standard chest or night table stands beside each unit, and there's a light over the head of the bed that can be turned on or off by the occupant. "There isn't even a place where I can cry!" one resident exclaimed.

In the wards, usually the residents of the beds nearest the window sills claim that area for their plants and flowers. Closet space in the form of metal cabinets, is normally along a third wall. Four straight-back chairs, one for each resident, make up the remainder of the room's furniture. A few nursing homes don't even have a divider or screens to give the occupant privacy for treatment or for dressing and undressing. Some are able to use the bathroom, but it is always a busy place, especially if someone has been given an extra laxative.

This kind of arrangement, mainly because of lack of space, prohibits seniors from bringing any possessions, such as their own TV, a favorite chair, lamp or pictures. If a senior doesn't like it, that's too bad; it's a seller's market and there's a waiting list for beds.

Seniors are no longer an invisible group. They are people, people with rights. They are human beings, and too often their humanness is lost in nursing homes and homes for the aged. Staffs of these institutions must be made more aware of the human side of their charges.

Dehumanization is due not so much to rising costs as to education—education of personnel. It costs less to care for happy seniors than unhappy ones who will create problems in morale or demand extra care if they retreat too deeply into themselves.

Can you imagine how a shy person feels when asked in front of a group of people, "Have you had a bowel movement today?" Or when that same person is half-naked and someone barges into their room, then leaves the door open when they go out? Talking over a resident's head as though he or she wasn't there is another demoralizing staff habit. "Residents also like to be hugged or have someone hold their hands, but they hate to be patted on the head like children," says Patricia Kinsella.

When seniors do adjust to institutional life, they hate to be shifted or have their routine broken; it upsets them greatly. When John developed a serious lung infection, he had to go to the hospital because the nursing home didn't have the facilities for treatment. He didn't recuperate as quickly as he should have, and his hospital stay went into its second week. When his family called the nursing home and said their father was well enough to return, the administrator said, "I'm sorry, John no longer has a bed here." Most homes have a time limit on holding a bed.

"What's he going to do?" they asked, shocked. "The hospital needs his room!"

Unfortunately, John's family could not find a vacancy at a home in the area, and because of pressure from the hospital, he was placed in a home 40 miles away. He knew no one, and friends couldn't visit easily. He died three months later—the emotional shock of not being wanted even in a nursing home was a contributing factor to the deterioration of his condition.

Nursing homes and homes for the aged still have a long way to go.

Forms and Legal Documents

Government and legal forms, because of their terminology, are frustrating and frightening to seniors. This apprehension is caused mainly by an education gap—a large number of today's seniors have only limited education. Completing grade eight was once considered sufficient education; finishing at grade three had to be accepted by others.

Over the last few years seniors have been drilled with "don't sign" advice: don't sign a contract, don't sign a power of attorney, don't—don't—don't! Instead of allaying their fears in this area, it has increased them. Our seniors were raised in an era when a man's word was his bond, when children looked after parents, when rights of inheritance were clear-cut. Times have changed and sound advice is needed, but it must be given with patience and understanding.

One of the best investments a senior can make for $25 to $75 is a will; it protects the ones you love.

Actually, it is not necessary to have a will. Under existing law, your wife or husband can still inherit the bulk of the estate. But what about grandchildren, or the old grandfather's clock you wanted to go to your niece? Unless your wishes are put down on paper, these relatives could end up with nothing. Whenever

135

money, property or other assets are involved, conflict over disposition too often comes into play.

The advantages of making a will are twofold: first, it enables the person to dispose of his or her estate as he/she sees fit, according to need, affection, duty or loyalty; second, the willor can choose someone he or she has confidence in to administer the estate.

When a person dies and there is no will, someone must apply to the court and formally ask for the job of administrator or executor. This can be a wife, son, daughter or good friend. If the court feels this person's application is not satisfactory, they can appoint someone else: a lawyer, trust company or public trustee.

A will does not necessarily have to be drawn up by a lawyer to be legal. It can be drawn up on a piece of tissue, but it must be *completely* handwritten by its maker with no printed matter of any description on the paper. This is called a holographic will. The law is very strict as to what it allows—the slightest bit of printed or typed material on a will is enough to disqualify it. A person cannot use a sheet of old letterhead from the office, hotel stationery, or the back of an envelope.

A handwritten will must be signed by you in the presence of two witnesses, and of course must be dated. Witnesses, though, cannot be beneficiaries. Even if a relative of a beneficiary is a witness, the gift becomes invalid. This is one point that must be clear: *witnesses cannot be beneficiaries or related to beneficiaries.*

There are a few states that allow a holographic will to be legal without having been witnessed. This, however, leads to litigation, even in states where it may be valid. Some states allow persons, under certain circumstances, to make an oral will; this, too, causes legal hassles later for many people.

Some people make out a will simply because they

don't want the government to get everything. This is a false assumption. In the United States, if the willor or testator, as that person is sometimes called, leaves more than a certain amount of property, both the state and federal governments will collect an estate tax. In Canada, the federal government eliminated the estate tax about four years ago.

Why should you appoint an executor? It is often easier if you appoint a lawyer, rather than a close friend or relative. Lawyers are experienced; they know exactly how to proceed. Also, if there are dissatisfied beneficiaries, they can cope more easily than a relative. An executor can be a wife, son, daughter, niece or nephew. The fees for the lawyer and the executor are taken from the estate; if the executor is a close relative, he or she usually declines a fee, taking only expense money. A trust company should always be involved if there is a considerable investment; they are better able to cope.

Insurance money simply goes to the beneficiary, unless the beneficiary is an estate. A wife does not have to declare insurance as income. If she invests it and receives interest, then the interest is taxable for the coming year; the initial gift is not.

A codicil is an amending paragraph which can be added to the will, or it can be a paragraph deleting a clause from the will without changing the whole document. To be legal, all codicils must be dated and witnessed. The codicil must be made according to state or provincial law, the same as the will.

Is money immediately frozen when someone dies? Yes, if bank accounts are over $5,000. However, if the deceased has six or seven bank accounts under $5,000, none of these will be frozen. Joint accounts are affected too, again, if the deposit is over $5,000. Unfortunately, this is not a set law in every state; it is, however, enforced in every part of Canada.

137

What about safety deposit boxes? An executor has the right to open and take out the will, nothing more! No investments can be touched. The executor must give a list of the box's contents to a supervising bank employee, and another list to the government agent. A release then comes back to the bank, and the executor can do with the contents as he has been instructed in the will, or as conscience directs.

What is probate? It is the Surrogate Court, and they must put their stamp of approval on the appointment of an executor. Whether or not the will needs to be probated depends on the size of the estate.

Sometimes, for reasons like suicide, there is a delay in settling an estate, although an executor is allowed just one year to distribute money and possessions, or otherwise "must show good reason" for such delay. In the meantime, beneficiaries can ask for interest on money.

The executor does have final say about burial and can overrule a will in this area. An executor also has the right to donate part of the body of the deceased for medical use.

Most dealings involving wills and estates are straightforward, unchallenged by courts and relatives, and range below the succession duty minimum. Wills are regarded as legal documents which act as a guide to the wishes of the deceased, and are treated with the respect that a person would desire.

Power of attorney is another type of legal document which involves seniors, and before being signed, these powers should be clearly defined.

A power of attorney can be limited or general in scope. General is very, very broad; in context, it takes over the running of another's life. Limited power, on the other hand, is delegated to certain areas or specific acts. The person receiving power of attorney does not have to be a lawyer; anyone can be appointed by a principal to this position.

Seniors need to be very careful about the person to whom they give this power. Most relatives or friends will consider it a trust and use it in the principal's best interest. A few will not—and therein lie the problems of greed and avarice, human failings which can attack even the best of us.

One senior gave her power of attorney to a niece; it was a limited one, with the trust company looking after her money. Maud, although she never told anyone, was afraid of her son-in-law, who could manipulate her daughter like a puppet. They lived in Maud's house almost rent free and sponged off her for food money when they ran short, although both had good jobs.

Maud had a cleaning lady, and later when the need arose, she had a live-in companion. She was quite happy at home, and since her health was good, the years ahead looked bright.

Then, one day the niece got a call from the trust company—they were sorry to hear Maud was failing and had been put into a nursing home (a very poor one) some distance from her own community.

"I've been on holidays and I haven't seen her for two weeks, but I'll check and get back to you," the niece said.

When she called Maud's daughter, she was informed that dear mother was just too much for any companion to look after, and after considering all the facts, the couple decided a nursing home was the best answer. They had also instructed that Maud receive no visitors because company would only upset her. The niece then called the family doctor; he said he didn't even know Maud had gone to a nursing home, and insisted that in view of her health and character, she should be home: "She'll be dead in a matter of weeks if she stays there."

The niece called the daughter. "Did you know that I have power of attorney for your mother?"

139

Astounded, the daughter angrily said she did not. Then the niece informed her that unless she removed her aunt from the nursing home and took her back to her own home, the niece would take the necessary legal steps and do it.

Maud was back in her own home the next day. She had lost 17 pounds. She hadn't eaten since she left home—she had just sat in a chair and cried. Even the nursing home administrator admitted, "She wouldn't have lasted long the way she was carrying on."

It took the 78-year-old woman several weeks to recover from her ordeal, but with a new companion, one who was interested in her needs, she was able to continue living at home for the next nine years. She died in her sleep, in her own bed, in her own home, the way she had always wanted to.

Almost as important as any document is a resumé of a person's important papers and where they can be located. Sometimes, at a time of great stress, a spouse is asked to make decisions, and the necessary papers can't be found. Or children who have been away from home for a long time may be called upon to act and have no idea as to the state of a parent's affairs.

Have documentation of all assets and liabilities on file. Then, in a safe place known to someone close to you, have the resumé of important papers and where they can be found.

If you need help in filling out forms, legal aid is available in most cities and towns across North America. If you're having problems with government forms, usually a representative will call at your home, or you can go to their nearest branch office.

And remember: government benefits are not paid automatically. You must apply on prescribed forms, and on certain claims there are time limits. Never, never put off applying for a benefit because you are frustrated by the forms. If you are eligible, it is yours by right.

Funerals for Seniors

To those who must stand by and watch, the coming of death often seems endlessly slow and painful. When death comes, funeral arrangements must be made, and the survivors are thrust into a situation saturated with quick decisions and high expense. Their grief is fresh and deep, and the only tangible way they have of expressing it is through the funeral service. Since it is the last thing survivors can do for the one who has died, they want the funeral to be the best money can buy, and too often they choose a service they can ill-afford.

Although prearranged funerals have been around for the last 30 years, growing public awareness of their affordability is just one of the reasons they are becoming a serious challenge to high-cost funerals. In a prearrangement situation, seniors are not under stress and can therefore make unhurried objective decisions. They feel freer to ask questions about cost, and if they like, they can comparison shop until they get the service that they feel would be most suitable for them.

There are other, more personal reasons for prearranging funerals. Often a spouse wants to make it

141

easier for the one left behind, or sometimes a senior has no relatives, or they live far away; both are sound reasons for working out a prearrangement.

All Canadian provinces have a Prearranged Funeral Act, and the Federal Trade Commission is working toward this end in the United States. Although specifics vary a bit from province to province and from state to state, the law basically protects the customer; if a funeral home goes bankrupt, the money is still safe. If interest has been building up for some time, the maximum a funeral home can take for administration costs is one-third of the interest up to a maximum of $100.

All money for prearranged funerals must, by law, be put into a trust fund in a liquid state (in such a way that it can be taken out within a few minutes). The interest on this money can accumulate and help defray the creeping costs of inflation, or it can be returned to the customer each year, leaving the principal the same. However, if someone has contracted for a $1200 funeral, they might now only receive $1000 service if the interest has been used.

Actually, a funeral is a ceremony which honors the memory and the body of the deceased and serves as a reminder that we will all pass this same way. Many ministers believe that funerals are primarily for the living, that their primary justification lies in the comfort and healing they can provide to grief-stricken relatives and friends.

Funerals are big business. Last year Americans spent $4 billion on funeral and burial arrangements, although funeral ceremonies are not required by law— they are simply our custom.

There are three types of funerals: the traditional, the disposal arrangement and the memorial service.

The traditional service involves about 80 hours of

142

work and covers such things as transportation, registration of death, medical and burial permits, services at funeral home, chapel or residence, embalming, casket, arrangement of flowers and acknowledgement cards.

Embalming is not mandatory, but unless specific instructions are received to the contrary, it is usually performed in the interest of preservation and sanitation.

The disposal arrangement is simply registration of death and burial permit, removal of the body from place of death, placing it in a plain, unlined container and transporting it to cemetery or crematorium.

A memorial service is held in memory of the deceased in a funeral home or a chapel. At these services there is no body—the burial or cremation has occurred at a different place and time. This service allows friends and relatives to express their respect for the deceased.

There are two ways of charging for a service: unit and functional. Unit pricing involves purchases of a whole package consisting of transportation, coffin, visitation and cars. With functional pricing, a funeral director charges for exactly what he or she does—if less is done, the charge is less. The casket, of course, is the biggest part of the funeral cost, and these costs vary a little from city to small town, depending on the area.

Payment for a funeral is expected within 30 days because directors must meet payroll and operating costs. But they are well aware that the liquid assets of an estate can be tied up for some time and they might have to wait. Where no funds are available, it is up to the municipality to see that "the man or woman, regardless of station in life, receives the dignity of a proper burial."

143

The purchase of a cemetery plot is separate from the funeral itself, although the director may, if desired, assist the family. Like everything else, cemetery plots have risen in price over the last few years. Now people are buying one plot and double- or triple-decking, which is perfectly legal. There is an extra charge of about $100 if pre-decking hasn't been arranged, or if the remains already in the grave have to be lowered. If the remains have only been in the ground a short time (one or two years) decking is not permitted. In England, cemetery plots can only be purchased for 14 to 21 years; in Canada it is a permanent purchase, as it is in most parts of the United States. Perpetual care, which is calculated into the price of the grave, is actually the yearly maintenance of the grave site.

Even though a spouse may own a plot, there is still a grave-opening fee, usually a flat fee set by the cemetery board. Now, with gravediggers unionized, many are charging extra for Saturday and Sunday grave openings.

In most areas cement liners are not required by law, but some cemetery boards, because of soil conditions, insist on them. These liners cost $200 and up.

In areas where the ground freezes early, remains are placed in a mausoleum in winter; later transfer to the cemetery is done at the convenience of the cemetery board and the funeral director, although the families are notified a day or two ahead. In the Arctic a body is usually frozen on a platform during the winter until burial can be performed in the spring.

Although it is possible to bury someone without the use of a funeral director, there are certain procedures that must be followed. The death must be registered by an immediate member of the family; it cannot be registered by a friend or neighbor, and a burial permit must be obtained from the registry office. The body must be placed into a container, which can even be a homemade box.

Both in the United States and Canada, less than .5% of all funeral services are performed without a clergyman. If the family does not have a minister, the funeral director will secure one. If the deceased has no church affiliation, an honorarium is put aside for the minister who attends. If the deceased has close ties with a particular church, usually there is no charge whatsoever.

Cremation has long been an accepted part of honoring the dead. In fact, there is evidence that cremation was used as far back as the Stone Age, and later by Greek and Roman civilizations. In many eastern countries the most common practice is to embalm the body and later cremate it with an elaborate ritual.

Cremation, though, has never been accepted by the Jewish people. Orthodox Jews bury their dead before sundown on the day of death, if possible. There is no embalming or dressing; the body is simply wrapped in a shroud. The funeral service is handled by a community burial committee and everyone is buried according to ancient traditions.

Cremation is becoming more common because of economic conditions, but if the family already has a plot, there is really not a great deal of difference in cost, so it boils down to a matter of choice.

Although cremation is on the increase in both Canada and the United States, it is still not widely accepted, except in certain areas. In other areas there may be no choice—in some parts of Canada and in the U.S. Midwest, crematoriums are nonexistent. In England, where facilities are abundant and there are limits on the term of traditional ground burial, the cremation rate is 70%.

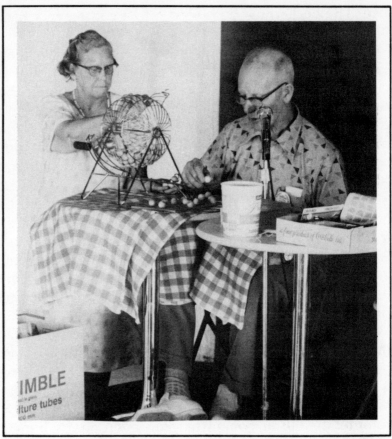

Lynda Middleton

Cremation charges average about $100 and the ashes can be left at the crematorium or placed in an urn or box which can then be buried in the family plot or scattered to the wind, if this is lawful in the area concerned. Many people are surprised to learn that the casket containing the body is also cremated, unless it is made of steel. In the United States, families can "rent-a-casket," but according to many funeral directors, the difference in cost does not yet compensate for the additional red tape involved.

There is no easy way to cut funeral costs, although memorial societies are taking a stab at it.

These societies act as a middleman; they help their members obtain a simple, dignified funeral by making arrangements with a particular funeral director at reduced prices because of the large number of people they represent. They do not perform funeral services.

The growth in the number of memorial societies has been slow and steady, with a sharp increase over the last few years. There are at present over 150 societies in the United States. In Canada, the British Columbia Society has 85,000 members, making it the largest in the world.

The goals of the society are simple. Through informative literature and other forms of communication, they offer an alternative to high-cost funerals. They provide a consulting service for members on all aspects of funerals, disposition of remains, types of observance and types of memorial service. They also encourage people to donate parts of their bodies to hospitals, and they serve as a watchdog on the funeral industry.

Membership in these memorial societies is open to anyone, regardless of race, color or creed. They are democratically run by a voluntary board of trustees and a limited paid staff. A one-time membership fee is $5 to $10, although some societies have a final "records charge" of $17 to $20. Although district societies are autonomous, the parent organization does receive 10% of all fees collected.

For those on fixed income, with little or no insurance, funerals can present a big financial burden. If possible, it is wise to start making contributions to pre-arrangement; otherwise, talk plainly without embarrassment to the funeral director about your financial status. Also, look at the alternatives offered through membership in a memorial society. Love and respect for the deceased come from the heart, not the purse.

Death and Dying

"To neglect, at any time, preparation for death is to sleep at our post; to omit it in old age, is to sleep during an attack."—Samuel Johnson.

For a long time, death and dying have been forbidden subjects; now they have been brought into the light of day. Death and dying are just as much a part of life's cycle as is birth, and it is time we put them into proper perspective.

The process of dying had an everyday familiarity to our grandparents; they died in their own homes surrounded by people they loved and who loved them. The young were not segregated from the old; both were integral to the family. Now seniors die in hospitals, nursing homes and homes for the aged, often with only staff members to hold their hand. Seventy-five per cent of all Americans die in institutions; in Canada statistics show that 70% die away from home.

Death for most of us is an abstract; we know it is inevitable, yet we push it away behind a curtain of silence. Madame De Staël, an 18th century French author, said, "We understand death for the first time when he puts his hand upon the one we love."

When bereavement comes, it can only be lived through. There is no way it can be made painless, but what we do beforehand can ease some of the problems facing those left behind.

"Burton always looked after our affairs," one woman said. "When I was left on my own, I didn't even know where the deed to our house was!"

Talking with your spouse about the future and the likelihood that one partner will have to go on without the other is not morbid, ghoulish or unlucky. It's plain common sense, and it's an expression of love—each is considering the future happiness of the other.

At a senior's workshop a man explained his fears: "I was always apprehensive about what would happen to Emma if I went first. Then one day we talked about it, and I was so relieved. Emma knows what she will have to face; she also knows how much money she will have, and she is prepared."

When someone we love dies, their problems are over, but those left behind, the spouse and the family, must go on living. Families should be encouraged to express their grief at the news of the death to come. Grievers usually go through many stages—restlessness, insomnia, self-reproach and lack of get-up-and-go, but anticipatory grief can be a cushion for the greater impact that is yet to come.

Our society has a natural inclination to conceal grief; we are afraid to let ourselves go. Grief should be felt; every attempt to divert it only extends the pain. The man or woman who has shared a life with someone for the last 40 years and has lost them needs to cry—suppressed emotion can bring on greater problems later. Research has shown that certain disorders, rheumatoid arthritis, asthma and in extreme cases, schizophrenia, can crop up if grief is not allowed to run its natural course.

Social activities like meeting friends and making conversation, mean nothing at this particular time. Don't expect chit-chat! Let the bereaved talk. According to Dr. Elliott Markham, psychiatrist at the New Mount Sinai Hospital, people should "just be good listeners and let the person in mourning reminisce if he or she wants."

People react differently to grief. One woman, when her mate died, removed every trace of him from their house. "Mother isn't human—she doesn't feel anything!" her children cried. She cared—she cared deeply, but this was her way of saying that this part of her life was over. She had to go on alone.

A few months later, a neighbor reacted in just the opposite way. He would not allow anyone to touch one thing of his wife's. Each day he put flowers in front of her picture; each night he turned down the bed for her.

The usual mourning period is eight to 12 weeks, and no binding decisions should be made, if at all possible, during that time. Usually, after three months some of that utter lostness is gone, although the grieving will continue for almost a year.

One man who remarried within three weeks later confessed, "It was the biggest mistake I ever made." It is natural to want a close relationship with someone else in the future, but emotions need time to adjust.

Some partners feel guilty when they feel relieved at the death of their spouse. Especially after a long illness, relief is natural—this glad-it-is-finally-over feeling is not a black cloud to be cast over a good relationship. The guilt feeling must be recognized for what it is, thankfulness that the person is no longer imprisoned in a pain-racked body.

There are untouched resources deep inside all of us; resources we can draw on when needed. Martha

150

was widowed less than a year ago. Although she was partially blind, she has learned to cope with the everyday challenges of living. "God never promised us a rose garden," she said, her hand searching for the plug of the electric tea kettle. "I'm lonely, and sometimes I'm afraid, especially at three or four in the morning, but later, when the dawn comes, my problems get back into proper perspective."

The best medicine for anyone who is mourning is to get away for a little while: travel, visit friends or stay with a relative. Just get away from the full impact of grief and those surroundings so full of memories and silence.

Some seniors must find a new meaning for life. Joan Crowther said, "When my husband died, I thought it was the end of everything. I wrapped the walls of my apartment around me like a security blanket."

Then one day she decided she just had to get going again. She became travel convener for a seniors building, and later took on the job of editor of a bi-monthly inter-building newsletter, which she found very rewarding.

As Joan learned, there is no better armor against loneliness and utter lostness than employment, paid or voluntary. Hiding oneself away behind closed doors is not going to solve anything.

Time is a healer, but it doesn't solve the problems; they still have to be faced by the bereaved. For weeks after the death of her husband, Mary's life had been in limbo. "Then one morning as I poured myself a cup of coffee, it suddenly hit me—I was alone, really alone!" For the first time in 42 years she was going to have to function without a partner. "I realized there wasn't anyone I could argue with except the dog, and he just pushed open the screen door and took off."

That morning Mary started to put her life back together again. She made a list of her assets and her liabilities, and when she was through she found she had three major problems facing her: money, a place to live and the need to retain a purpose for living. She and her husband had lived all their lives within a nine-mile radius of where they were born.

Jack, who was 68 when he died, had been receiving a government old-age pension and Mary had been receiving the spouse's supplement. Now even this was ended.

Shortly after the funeral a government representative came to see her. She assured him that despite the loss of the pension, she was going to be all right.

But when all the bills were in, an entirely different picture emerged. There was the insurance money, but that was only $1,000; Jack had had rheumatic fever when he was a boy and it had left him with a heart problem that had made coverage more expensive.

The insurance had been a bugbear for Mary. In every conversation the agent had assured the family, "If anything goes wrong, you'll have the money in a matter of days." That had been a myth. After five letters and numerous telephone calls, the check finally came. "I swear it took the scenic route via the Orient," Mary told her daughter.

This wasn't the only problem she had come up against. There was "the will Jack was always going to have drawn up and didn't." As if Mary didn't have enough worries, her neighbor had patted her hand in sympathy and said, "Oh my dear, the government will just step in and take everything!"

This, fortunately, wasn't true. The estate had been immediately turned over to the family lawyer and in a few weeks everything had been transferred to Mary's name.

The years had not always been kind to the couple; they had worked hard, but they never had gained much financially. Their whole lives had been tied up in their family and farm. With Jack gone, the farm now became a problem. Mary could rent the land to give her income, but the house was big. "It costs a fortune just to heat it," Mary said, "and besides, it needs a family—not a lonely old widow wandering around its empty rooms."

"Why don't you build yourself a small cottage?" her son-in-law asked her. "Take a half-acre off that cornfield; that would make an excellent lot and you would be living right here in your own community." Some of the family had been advocating that she move into a high-rise in the nearest town.

Her son-in-law's suggestion made sense. The money from the sale of the farm would solve her financial problems. A cottage on the corner lot would be just the right size for her, and close, yet not too close, to her family. She would still be living in the community she knew and loved.

Building on that corner lot seemed the ideal solution. It was—until they tried to get the lot severed from the main part of the farm, and then Mary slammed head-on into regional planning. "There is just no way you can get permission to sever that lot!" the township clerk told her.

Even though it was still foreign to her, she had a new role as a widow—she had to fight for herself. "You mean I can't keep a small piece of land for myself!" she stormed. "For the last 42 years my husband and I paid taxes; sometimes we had to go without basics just to do it. If anyone in this community needed help, we were there with whatever we had. Now I need a place to live, a place to build a cottage, and you dare sit there and tell me I can't!"

When she appeared before the planning board, it was also adamant—no severance. She appealed its decision and was later granted the necessary permission.

"She would never have been content in a housing complex, and this seemed the only solution," a councilor was heard to say after the appeal. Mary's story had a happy ending.

There are many myths and half-truths that seem to be linked to death and the bereaved; one misconception is that a widower, after a few respectful months of mourning, is a happy-go-lucky, carefree fellow, literally deluged with invitations. Actually a widower's life is quite the opposite, at least for most. They are lonely, unhappy, frustrated and consider themselves fortunate to be invited to make a fourth for bridge.

Widowers get short-changed too, especially in the area of benefits. The American Council of Life Insurance says that widowers receive only 4% of all benefits paid through life insurance. Widows receive the bulk of benefits (54%), mainly due to the fact they live longer than their husbands. The other 42% is divided among children, partners, employees, trusts, institutions and estates. On the rare occasion when an eccentric leaves his or her benefits to a dog or cat, this becomes part of the 42%.

Many books of advice have been written to guide the widow, but few have been written to guide the widower. Why? As the male of the species, he is traditionally supposed to be better able to cope than this wife if she were to survive him, and the widower is simply less visible—there are five widows to every widower.

"Charlie will be all right. He will remarry," friends and neighbors said when Louise died. They

154

usually made sure that Charlie, in a discreet way of course, could hear them. "Men can handle these things better than women!"

Can they? It's true they don't shed as many visible tears (tears aren't masculine, people say, a myth in itself), but widowers cry just as much, maybe more, on the inside. Tears are a vent to our emotions; if we smother them, they are just going to rise up in another form, probably more explosively, later on.

Work is the best antidote we have for bereavement. Charlie returned to his part-time job as custodian at the library the week following the funeral. Being around people and working helped him keep his mind off his grief, but it was the solitary times that really got to him.

His children had been good; for the first few weeks they invited him for supper and paid more than the occasional visit to his home, but they had their own lives to live, and Charlie knew he had to pick up the threads of his own.

"It's the little joe-jobs that really get to me," he told his friend Hodge. "I'm always yanking off a button, and now there's no one to sew it on."

Breakfast turned out to be another problem for Charlie. He always read the paper, and Louise always complained. Now he didn't even bother to read it— the incentive was gone. He had always enjoyed those verbal skirmishes.

Up to now Charlie had also enjoyed eating; now he didn't care if he ate or not. "When I used to come home, no matter what crazy hours I was working, Louise would have a meal ready, and a pre-dinner drink waiting on the mantel."

When Charlie comes home these days, he has to make his own meal and mix his own drink, and that's where another problem has emerged. He not only mixes one drink, he mixes two, sometimes three or four, and he forgets to eat altogether.

Even the laundry has taken on a different dimension now. After Louise died, his daughter had taken care of his dirty clothes, but she has three children and a part-time job too, and Charlie feels this was imposing on her time. He would do his own—nothing to it! Just throw the clothes in the automatic, pour in some detergent, push the button and when the cycle was finished, toss the whole mess into the dryer and forget it. That's exactly what he did, forgot it until he needed a clean shirt. He hauled it out of the dryer, and instead of it being clean and fresh, it looked more like a cleaning rag. And the white things—instead of being white like those in TV commercials, they were sticky and gray.

"Why don't you get yourself a nice widow woman?" asked his friend Hodge, who listened to his complaints.

Charlie had toyed with the idea, but it had been 38 years since he had asked anyone for a date. There were a couple of women who had been more than friendly—should he send flowers, or, like in his day, just call with a box of candy in hand?

But Charlie had a problem that no one knew anything about—he still felt married to Louise. It was true that in their vows they had said "until death us do part," but the contract for him was still valid. In his heart he was still bound to his wife.

Gerontologists tell us that people whose lives intertwine, like Charlie and Louise, suffer most from the death of a spouse. Especially in later years, each should develop some area of interest apart from the other so that if one is left, he or she still has a portion of life to continue with, free of the infringement of memories.

Ed Heal/The London Free Press

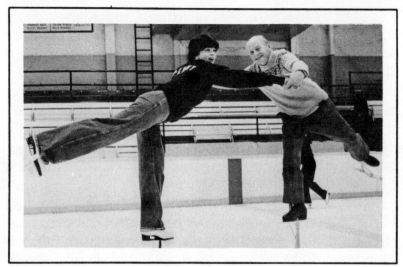

Death of a spouse in a marriage where there is a pattern of over-dominance leaves the greatest void. If the dominant one dies, the other has no leader; if the passive one dies, the dominant one has no one to lead or bully.

Terminal illness is hard to take, but it is worse if the family can't talk. Every word, every phrase is guarded because it might be taken out of context.

When Marsha first learned that her husband Frank was terminally ill with cancer, she said, "I went around like a zombie. I moved—I did all the things I was supposed to do, said all the things I was supposed to say, but I wasn't feeling. All my emotions were tied into a tight knot."

One day, after a "crying jag," she realized she and Frank had just quit communicating; there was no closeness between them anymore. "That monster was always there. I remembered the nurse telling us that we should get the subject out into the open, so I spoke to Frank about the cancer. It was like a load being lifted off our shoulders as we both accepted the inevitable."

Dr. Elisabeth Kübler-Ross, psychiatrist and author of *Death and Dying*, feels patients should be told they are dying. If they are denied this knowledge they cannot summon their emotional strength.

Some patients want to know how they are going to die—will they just slip away in their sleep, or will the end be long and painful? Most want to die with dignity. If they can't discuss this because they're not supposed to know about their condition, more stress is placed upon them.

John had an illegitimate son who was partially handicapped. For years he had secretly been contributing to the boy's welfare. Now he was dying and he wanted to make sure this financial assistance would continue. He didn't want to spell it out in his will, yet he wanted the boy protected. John needed to talk to someone, to say, "Hey, listen—I'm dying, and I want to know what to do about Billy."

As it turned out, his wife had always known about her husband's illegitimate son, and she was quite prepared to see that the financial support for the boy continued. Had they talked (John only made his confession a few hours before he died), his final weeks would have been much easier.

People who are terminally ill should never be made to feel that all hope is gone. They must have a thread to hold onto, although this does not mean extending false hopes and dreams of a miracle. When a senior "just gives up," death is usually not far away.

No one really understands how a dying person feels—we haven't yet had the experience. Dying is a putting together of all we've been—the sum total of our lives.

Often the closest people to someone who is dying are the staff of the hospital. Nurse's aides, even the cleaning people, often have a more natural intimacy with the dying than some who are called professionals. But now the medical and social sciences are bringing the whole family unit into this process of death, dying and bereavement with palliative care, a new term that simply means quality care for those soon to die. The care of the terminally ill and dying has been sadly neglected by many professional people because even doctors and nurses shy away from death and dying.

Now, along with palliative care, have come hospices, places where those who are dying can find peace instead of denial in their surroundings, a place where they can die with dignity. In medieval days, a hospice was a way station offering shelter and rest to weary travelers.

According to the latest figures from Washington, about $2.5 million has been provided as seed money for local hospices. In Canada two years ago a palliative care unit of 30 beds was set up at Montreal's Royal Victoria Hospital, a two-year pilot project of the Quebec Department of Social Affairs. Since then, palliative care units have opened in Vancouver, Winnipeg, Windsor and Toronto.

"We try to think of the hospice as admitting the whole family rather than just the patient," says Dr. Cicely Saunders, medical director at St. Christopher's Hospice in London, England, which is looked upon as a model throughout the world.

There are two major areas where palliative care can help a patient: it can relieve them of pain, and it can provide their remaining days with the best in supportive care so that the dying person's life retains its quality right to the end.

Death may be the last great mystery and misery, but we have nothing to fear so long as we act from our hearts in our care for the dying and those who remain.